The Sun Shines Through

How to Save Your Own Life
(and other misadventures)

The Sun Shines Through

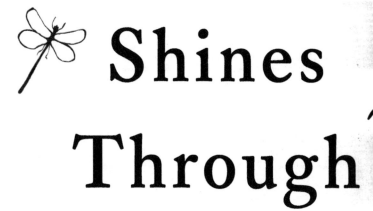

The Story of Two Cancers
and Cannabis Oil

Sharon King

The Book Guild Ltd

First published in Great Britain in 2019 by
The Book Guild Ltd
9 Priory Business Park
Wistow Road, Kibworth
Leicestershire, LE8 0RX
Freephone: 0800 999 2982
www.bookguild.co.uk
Email: info@bookguild.co.uk
Twitter: @bookguild

Typeset in 11pt Minion Pro

Printed and bound in the UK by TJ International, Padstow, Cornwall

ISBN 978 1912881 970

British Library Cataloguing in Publication Data.
A catalogue record for this book is available from the British Library.

To Jasper, who taught me how to love and how to let go.
To family and friends, who helped me to find my way back.

What follows is a true account of love and loss, and the use of cannabis oil to treat lung cancer (his) and breast cancer (hers). Spanning the years 2012 to 2019, this memoir recalls the lives of a married couple, both diagnosed in the same year, and their attempts to save their own lives.

Who We Were

People have asked me, "Does this story have a happy ending?" What can I reply? I haven't got there yet.

I have learnt so much over recent years:

How to be patient, endlessly. How to be a patient.

How to sit for hours, for lifetimes, waiting for outcomes.

I have learnt how to be still, how to quell fear and longing, how to reside alongside grief in its many forms and faces. How to live and be a part of a picture that is broken, sore and compelling. How to accommodate loss, live carefully amongst it and defer it at times, so it does not pull me under at every turn.

Love can be compared to a needle and thread; it sews us together and binds us. It is also a needle so sharp; it stabs us with longing and loss, in expected and wholly unexpected ways, but it still holds strong through its rips, tears and pulls; it cannot be undone.

We, the bereaved, reside in that place between night and day. Imagine being on a flight and looking out the tiny window at the sun setting over a high horizon; above the line the sky is red, through orange, yellow and blue; underneath it there is only

1

darkness. The grieving live within the line. Sometimes we soar above in the orange, yellow and blue, carried by memories and hope. Mostly we live below, in the darkness of the cloud. As life goes on, as surely it must, we learn to fly higher, to seek the light, to pull the threads tight and take our lives and our loss and our memories with us.

I have begun to hope for a happier ending. I am willing to consider it and hope that it is not too greedy of me to want it. I have been gifted with so much love already; I cannot complain if that's all there is. These days I am lighter in heart and spirit; the sun shines through.

Here is our story

This is not an easy story to write. Death and widowhood are challenging subjects. Cancer is ugly, cruel and dark, but maybe you know that already.

In amongst the extreme challenges that cancer always brings, there is also humour, beauty and grace. We often found ourselves laughing out loud at our dark humour. We found joyous moments of pure understanding; understanding of the human condition, and that we, and the world, are beautiful. Life became precious as the irrelevancies of day-to-day life and the tiny, silly stresses disappeared. And then there is grace; grace under pressure. There is grace in the face of pain beyond measure.

I was inspired to write it – perhaps driven is a better phrase – after reading Joyce Carol Oates' *A Widows Story*, which is a stream of consciousness about her experiences as an 'unexpected' widow. I read it over an intense forty-eight hours, as I tried to fill another weird, lonely week in November 2015, and found myself becoming animated for the first time in three years, or more. I had clarity of thinking; I would try to articulate, I would try to exorcise some of my experience, and in doing so perhaps I could begin to clear the way to my healing and to becoming a creative again, as I used to be: a poet, a writer, a wordsmith, a songstress. Maybe it could help me come back to being a functioning person.

I have used a mixture of memories, diary entries and Facebook posts to try and weave a timeline through the years. Looking back through my scant diary entries over the first half of this 'journey' I am bewildered at what I find; I am like a clumsy detective, scrabbling around for clues in the bottom drawer of my memory. The diary entries, particularly the few early ones, are the worst of me – why would I publish them?

Some days I feel I am the only still person at a busy junction or train station. I stand waiting, while all around me, in triple time, the crowds move and surge, a fast ebb and flow of humanity. I have no understanding of why, or how, and in writing this I hope to find some peace.

Cannabis oil played its part in our story. Its medicinal use in the Western world is a new science, still in its infancy as we began our journey in 2013. However, for many centuries it has been used in its natural plant form for healing, in both Native American and Eastern philosophies. Marijuana was only outlawed in America in the early 1900s when the medical model split between the new-style physicians and old-fashioned healers.

I hope our experience of cannabis oil will aid general understanding of its uses, its benefits and its pitfalls. It must be acknowledged that cannabis oil is not a panacea. There are over two hundred different cancers, all with their own particular devious ways of ruining a body and mind, and for some people cannabis oil may not be an appropriate treatment. I do not hold a position of whether it can help everyone. I am only relating what it meant for us. However, I do believe its healing properties are most beneficial when the oil is used in conjunction with an organic, alkalising diet, as described later in this book.

I can't begin our tale without some background on who we once were. It's so long ago, in both space and time, that it's almost impossible to recall our old life. We had been together sixteen years before we were diagnosed. Jasper became stepdad to my seven-year-old daughter and married me shortly after we met in 1997, when he moved from Sheffield into my house in Edinburgh as my lodger. We fell madly and beautifully in love within six weeks of his arrival. I was thirty years old; he was twenty-six. We were fragile, in our own ways; Jasper had lost his mum to cancer when he was only ten years old, my first boyfriend Keith died when I was fifteen. I also had a catastrophic motorbike accident at age eighteen, which damaged my pelvis so badly, I was advised, after my daughter was born by elective caesarean section in 1990, that I could have no more children. We had also experienced difficult times in our previous relationships, and as we fell in love we talked openly about our need for honesty, loyalty, gentleness and joy. We were best friends, soulmates; we could speak across a room without talking; our friends loved our love and took inspiration from it too. We were happy.

Our wedding party, in September 1999, was held in a field near Coldingham, and was a three-day event. We persuaded and cajoled our far-flung community to help in any way they could. NoFit State Circus provided a large big top for cost; our friends and relatives were given a workshop in how to raise such a beast and take it down again. Simple Simon Catering provided our wedding meal and breakfast for cost. Our sound engineers, Dave and Tim, worked all weekend, not even for cost. Stewart provided our PA and backline, and Edward II and Mystery Juice performed for us. DJ Dolphin Boy kept us up all night with a six-hour set. We camped, danced, ate and celebrated. Our community came together, with love, to make it happen. It was a joyous event and the sun shone all weekend.

We were performers; songwriters, wordsmiths, musicians, jugglers and raconteurs. He was successfully travelling the world with his theatre company. I struggled as a singer-songwriter at grass-roots level, happy and creative, but always working very hard to keep my head above water here in the UK. When we were together, in other words not on tour or gigging, which was about a third of the year at that time, we were active people. Jasper loved golf, snooker, darts, football and walking. We especially loved exploring the local beaches in East Lothian, and on the west coast of Scotland and our beloved island of Eigg.

In the spring of 2012, we had both been granted residency visas in Australia. As a regular visitor and performer in the country Jasper had his entry visa stamped in summer 2012, and I was planning an Australian tour in February 2013 to complete the process. It was a new beginning, a possible new life for us, although we really hadn't decided. We saw it as an opportunity to live and work in the country for a while, still coming back to the UK and mostly living and working here. We had a wide community in Australia, and I had family there. We were full of dreams to buy a bit of land and set up a home and garden.

We were happy here in Scotland but bored with our lives. We had a large and varied group of friends; locally in our city of Edinburgh, across the wider UK and in Australia. Although very successful in his field, my husband was tired of the constant travelling and living away from home that his job entailed, and was considering a complete change of direction into care work.

He would have been very good in this vocation; he was a very caring man, with a humorous, cheeky, gentle manner. He won over everyone he met. He saw it as a challenge to raise a smile from folks – the grumpy butcher around the corner from the flat, the salesperson, the postman; whoever he encountered – and generally he did just that. I was happy in my work, beginning to get noticed by the industry and the public, and finally I was beginning to reap some rewards for my many years of hard graft.

I was distracted through the spring and summer of 2012. I had been awarded a Quality Production Grant by Creative Scotland that would allow me to produce my fourth album in a well-respected studio. I worked every hour of the day and then some; writing, creating, rehearsing and marketing my new product. It went live in July and the summer was a whirl of album releases, gigs and radio promotions.

However, in amongst this hive of activity there was already a backdrop of unease. I guess the first time I can remember thinking *something's not OK with Jasper* was at a friend's birthday weekend in May 2012. Jasper had become breathless and listless; he had a slight yet persistent cough. He had been feeling depressed and had not been his normal positive self for quite some time. I pushed him to attend the local GP surgery and he was told he had a chest infection and was given antibiotics. Things didn't improve. But since he had recently gone through a vigorous medical for his Australian visa, he felt anything sinister would have been picked up in that process.

Meanwhile we were also involved with the care and support of a close friend who had, two years previously, been diagnosed with cancer. Mim was single, with no family close by, and she was very reliant on friends to help her through her rounds of surgery, chemotherapy and radiotherapy. I was involved in helping a bit with her day-to-day needs, as well as supporting her best friend Suzy while she supported Mim. 'Distracted' is the right description. Maybe if I had had my eye more firmly on my husband I could have made more of a difference. Useless rumination, I know. But still, these questions haunt me. They have become a part of my 4am panic into wakefulness.

By September, Mim was very poorly and we were constantly back and forth visiting her in the hospice. Meanwhile, Jasper was getting worse. He saw the GP again and was sent for a chest X-ray. Warning bells were ringing loudly in my head when the surgery called shortly after to say he needed another one. The previous X-ray had shown some signs of inflammation which they needed to treat again with antibiotics.

Mim died in the hospice in November 2012, and as she left us, our friends were already noticing what couldn't be hidden any longer. Jasper was very unwell. I will never forget being at the hospice for Mim's last days and Suzy quizzing me about Jasper and asking us both, "What's really going on?"

Through November and December, he had endless tests at the local teaching hospital for a possible diagnosis of a respiratory disease called sarcoidosis, a condition that we researched and were terrified to think he might have. I was privately very afraid it was cancer, but I kept these fears largely to myself; we alluded to it together, but we laughed off our fears as ridiculous. In hindsight, we should have been referred immediately to the cancer unit in Edinburgh, or at least much sooner than we were. I don't understand why we were seen at the general hospital. It seemed so obvious to me. All his symptoms pointed to lung cancer.

All through that sad autumn of Mim's passing and on through the build-up to Christmas and Hogmanay we kept our own counsel. We told no one of our fears and pretended to friends and family we had it all under control, we were not that worried. Privately we both knew it was big, and regularly discussed how utterly terrified we were. We struggled with cash; Jasper could not work, he was already too unwell, and as a self-employed person this meant no pay, and as there was no diagnosis we were not entitled to extra help from the government. Our sex life, which had always been active and fun, had dwindled to zero; we talked about it openly and tried to invent ways to get our mojo back. We didn't realise this was also a symptom.

We went out dancing as the year turned – a huge night out for Hogmanay, as ever – and now in retrospect I think he knew this would be his last big party. Jasper had a lung biopsy in very early January. By now, we were just waiting for the bomb to drop that would tear our lives apart. It arrived in early January and was worse than either of us had had the capacity to imagine.

How on Earth Did We Get Here?

13th January 2013

"I'm sorry to inform you, Mr King, that you have Stage 4 lung cancer, with spread to the lymph nodes and bone. The cancer is inoperable and incurable. However, you are one of the lucky 10%" (*Lucky? Lucky?!*) "and you may well respond to a targeted gene therapy called Tarceva (erlotinib). This *may* prolong your life by up to two years, possibly longer."

We sit in the consultant's office, stunned beyond words, shocked beyond measure. How can this be true? We have known for quite a few months something is wrong: increased breathlessness, tiredness, a shallow cough. All the signs are there; looking back, it's so obvious. After all, he has been increasingly unwell since the previous spring. Cancer has slid into our lives, slowly, imperceptibly, almost unnoticed, but not quite. It has been there all along, deep in our psyches; we knew it without knowing. It presents as a lack of joy, a slipping into depression, sleeplessness and a panic that seems to have no ground or reason.

"How long, if the Tarceva doesn't work?" I ask.

"Four months," the consultant replies.

This moment is frozen in time for me. I cannot imagine not knowing it, in all its awful detail, and I am sure it will stay with me till my end of days. Everything moves in slow motion and my eyes are on Jasper's face. The consultant is patient, she sits quietly waiting, while we try, we strain and attempt to 'hear' what she has said.

The body shock, the trembling, the rapid movement through the scales of emotion is profound, too fast to catch hold of. It is caught in a freeze frame, this moment of discovery. Life stops here, business cancelled, all on hold. My legs feel like rubber, and this doesn't stop for over six months.

Jasper was officially declared unfit for work, and under DWP special rules (expected to live less than six months) he was signed onto the highest level of disability. I cancelled my tour to Australia. However, the entry visa official, who was fan of my husband's work, was very helpful and gave me an extension on my entry time to the following November. Everything was in flux. I formally mothballed my business at the beginning of February 2013 and became my husband's full-time carer. We agreed we would spend as much time together as we could. I had one more tour to honour through July, and some autumn gigs planned, but we decided we would cross those bridges when they came.

First Facebook post, 20th January 2013

Dear friends, the response to our news this week has been overwhelming. Thank you. For those who are unaware, Jasper had a lung biopsy recently and it has been confirmed that he has a primary tumour on his upper right lung. It's a non-small-cell adenocarcinoma.

We have very little other information at present. He has another scan on Tuesday to check if there is spread, and possibly another biopsy the week after. We will then know better what we are dealing with and our treatment options. So, in two or three weeks we should have more info to share with you.

Folk keep asking what they can do, practically speaking. We both believe very much in the healing power of positive thought. So, please keep us in your hearts and send us your positive, healing thoughts when you can.

Please also 'like' and share this post. We are very keen to reach the many strands of our community across the world and maximise this positive energy, while also letting folks know the info we have. I know there's not much to like and it seems absurd, but it will keep the status current and help keep that positive, healing energy flowing.

Jasper is his usual smiley, positive self and, although exhausted, is doing well. Please feel free to message either of us. We really do value your support and love and we will always try to respond. If you don't hear back from us, though, don't worry. We are quite overwhelmed at times, and incredibly tired.

That's it, really; we are shocked and terrified, of course. But we know we will get through this with the support and love of our friends. It may seem a contradiction to be both positive and terrified, but the maelstrom of emotions swing so fast and it is possible to feel both.

In the meantime, it's business as usual, as much as is possible, so please keep in touch. Folks are wondering about the practical work aspect for the next few months. The company will be working as normal, with a deputy for Jasper. I will also be working as normal, although the Australian tour – starting in two weeks – is going to need some amending! Australian pals, I will be in touch very soon.

More info when we have it. All our love to you.

Sharon and Jasper. xxxx

We were devastated and reeling. There were no words of comfort, no solutions, no way out. I began my grieving then. I came home and I wept and railed, and wept and railed, for many months. I did not want to live. Friends gathered; family gathered. We sat inside our shock. Jasper began the Tarceva immediately and for a few months we went through all seven bells of hell while he acclimatised to the drug. This awful, precious, life-prolonging drug ravaged his skin with infected boils and dreadful sore rashes and caused horrible infections in his eyes and under his nails. The Tarceva caused his hair to become very brittle. His eyelashes grew extraordinarily long, but some also grew inward, causing much pain and discomfort. I hated to see what it was doing to his body, and I feared what was happening to his stomach and bowel. But it worked, it slowed the cancer, and we settled into a horror of waiting. I rallied and began to research options. I put us on a strict diet of all-organic, alkalising foods, and water, water, so much water. We were juicing a pound of carrots per day and drinking dreadful green juices that made us want to vomit. I was working so hard to save him. I felt it must be possible. We could do it. Our love would win through.

Facebook post, 22nd February 2013

Words have been so hard to find these past six weeks or so. THANK YOU comes easy though: to all who have come when we called, contacted us, caught us, sent love, sent flowers, sent carrots, sent holidays, sent gifts, sent positive thoughts and sent cures. WOW – we have been truly overwhelmed.

Here is where we are at. Jasper's cancer is an advanced adenocarcinoma; it is Stage 4, primary to his lung, and there is secondary spread through his lungs, lymph nodes and rib bones. The oncologist believes it to be incurable. We believe in the power of thought and love.

He began treatment yesterday with targeted chemo – Tarceva – which he takes every day in pill form. This will hopefully stop the spread and may even reduce the tumour's size. We are also creating a world of health with many, many, many carrots and other fruit and vegetables in an amazing juicer we were gifted. We have great ongoing care and advice, from both oncology and our very own Susana.

Jasper is basically 'well', and although very easily tired and sometimes breathless, he is really doing fine. He needs lots of rest, the best organic nutrition, and he simply cannot catch a cold or flu. We are adjusting slowly to the huge changes, learning to live more in the moment and to enjoy the important things in life; family, friends and love. We laugh a lot and I cry sometimes.

Please keep us in your thoughts and prayers, and if you come to visit, bring a smile with you and please leave your coughs and colds at home. If we don't answer the phone, the doorbell or emails, it's not because we don't want to hear from you. It's quite simply that we are exhausted or need to have a bit of time to ourselves. Or we may even be out living it up! So please do keep trying. xxxxx

We decided very early on to attend our local Maggie's Centre, to ask for advice and to try to find some peace within ourselves. We initially hated the place. It represented too much for us. It made our situation much too real. We persevered though, as I was particularly aware that there might come a time when we really needed them. I imagined myself walking in, on some future far-off date, and falling to the floor in a sobbing mess, and then they would already know me, they would understand. I wouldn't have to begin at the beginning of our story. They would scoop me up and help me.

Maggie's Centre proved to be invaluable for us over the years. The highly skilled and knowledgeable staff supported us at every turn, and we received regular expert advice, care and counselling. I watched them clear the decks for Jasper when I took him there one day, many, many months later; he was almost catatonic with toxicity due to claustrophobia and his medication: anti-nausea, antidepressants, Valium, Tarceva and slow-release morphine pills all creating a huge payload within his body. The Maggie's staff immediately organised a psych assessment and spoke to his Marie Curie doctors about reducing the huge amounts of medication. They were interested in our wish to use cannabis oil, and they tried to support us as much as they could with our decisions regarding different treatments. For over two years, I attended a regular Monday support group for carers of terminally ill partners and, although it was a gruelling weekly event that often created much fear in me for what lay ahead, it also provided me with a vital outlet for my own grief and stress. It was a safe place to say, "I hate this, I can't do this", with no judgement. I still attend Maggie's for one-to-one bereavement counselling, and I am so very grateful and glad I have that incredible resource to access. I would encourage anyone facing a cancer diagnosis to try and attend their local centre. Get to know the staff, get past the initial difficulty. They can really make a huge difference, if only as a safe and comfortable place to regroup in between hospital appointments and treatments. Maggie's operates on an open-door drop-in policy and there's always a welcome and a cup of tea from folks who know what strain you may be under, be it as a patient or a family member.

I don't remember much of the first half of 2013, six unspeakable months of grief, fear, panic, sleeping pills, a minefield of erratic emotions and deep loneliness; all crushing in their absoluteness. I cried hard, long and alone, in the nights, while he slept through. We were together but apart somehow, and we were facing the knowledge that this was our new truth; we are all alone really.

We also laughed and joked and pretended we were OK, because what else could we do? We kept on keeping on. We sheltered in each other's arms. I fell apart while he remained mostly upbeat and definitely in denial. He would often say to people that it was worse for me than him because I would have to stay here after he had gone, I didn't agree with him. Jasper had very few cancer symptoms; he was breathless and tired, but apart from that, you would never know he had a death sentence hanging over him. It was incredibly strange to live this half-life, it was surreal, and the shock waves went on and on and on. So strong, the physical shock to the body. Wow, who could know it could go so deep and take so much from a person?

The biggest challenge? To stay alive. For him, the battle with the invading cancer, which he fought with calm dignity and grace, and for this, I loved him more.

For me? To stay alive. To fight the invading darkness, to somehow learn to reach out and make the call, if only to say, "Please share this moment with me. It's too big, I'm going under."

I realised through that first spring that a portion of the anxiety, panic, breathlessness and wobbly legs I was experiencing was being fuelled by an addiction to sleeping pills. Zopiclone is a powerful and addictive drug and should only be used short term, a couple of weeks at the most. I had been on it for six months. The pills also, curiously, exaggerated the sensations in the tip of my tongue when I was in withdrawal, and this would become quite maddening. I stopped using zopiclone and instead opted for occasional nights using a mixture of diazepam and temazepam. However, these pills also have a 'hangover' effect and can help fuel a 4pm teary meltdown. I have now developed a healthy respect for the fact that pills are short-term props. One or two nights every few weeks is fine, but any more than that can have a profound effect. A small amount of cannabis oil is a much better sedative and can guarantee a good eight hours' sleep if it's taken a couple of hours before bedtime. Taken too late it can have the opposite effect and cause restlessness, anxiety and lack of sleep.

What an incredibly, indescribably lonely time for us both; the spiral into ill health and an incurable, inoperable diagnosis, and a sentence of very limited time; four to eight months prognosis. Before our life was shattered, we had been very sociable, regularly hosting dinner parties for fourteen folks or more in our large, sunny, Victorian tenement flat. Hogmanay would be brought in with a big celebratory meal at ours for whoever arrived. We would see the bells in at home and then head out to a party. There were a few years where I would make a pie that could stretch to twenty-five folk, and regularly did. Our large flat was also the hub for many after-after-parties, and often a big night out clubbing would find us greeting the dawn back at ours; dancing, singing, loving, laughing and living.

Through that early time, I was completely traumatised by my anticipatory grief and my crushing fear of losing Jasper. In the background I also had my own realisations: I too was possibly quite ill. It's very hard to remember anything about those early months. I wrote nothing during that time, or in fact for the following six months; there are no diary entries, no creative words or songs. I was struck dumb for the first time ever. Jasper was generally stoical, and although he was regularly poorly with the Tarceva side effects of constant skin and nail infections, he was in no pain. He seemed mostly happy, which drove me crazy as I couldn't understand why he wasn't in a mess like me. I realised, of course, it was just his way of outwardly coping. But we both suffered terribly with loneliness, despite our friends trying to reach across the divide to us. Every day was lived in limbo, never looking more than four months ahead, living within our restrictions; emotional, mental, physical and spiritual.

Facebook post, 26th July 2013

A good result today from oncology, Jasper's tumours are static, and we don't have to go back for three months. Let's have some summer fun and stop to smell the roses. xxx

Another Cancer...

In July of the same year (probably earlier, now I understand better the insidious nature of this clever disease), I realised the lump in my right breast was not going away. It was growing, and my skin was puckering. I too had cancer. But how could that be true? How could we both be afflicted? It made no sense to my exhausted and stressed brain, and so I kept my secret; I told no one, as I knew that, as soon as I did, I would have to deal with it. We would have to deal with it.

I honoured the final tour with my band in July 2013, but I was bone-weary, traumatised and deeply frightened. The tour was a nightmare and cost me a couple of thousand pounds in wages and accommodation fees. I had not received the funding I had applied for because my funding application was very weak. It was written in haste and with little care, as our world collapsed around us. I had applied for funding to tour far-flung places, taking original music to remote village halls across the Highlands and Islands. It was tour that depended on funding; a tour that was never going to make money; a tour that would always be played to very small communities. Jasper and I spoke every morning and night on the phone. Every day I was away, I felt that I was moving in the wrong direction. My every instinct was to run for home and hold my man while I could. He told me on the phone one night, after a particularly soul-destroying gig on South Uist playing to a handful of people, that he was scared the cancer had spread to his brain. I knew I must be crazy, honouring a tour that no one cared about, driving in completely the wrong direction, heading further north when I needed to be bolting south for home. I sang and played my guitar every night to small crowds, while the growing lump in my breast pressed painfully against the body of the guitar. It interrupted my normally relaxed banter and my concentration, and never gave me a minute's peace.

I arrived home in late July, utterly broken, all confidence in myself and my music gone. I was £2,000 in the red and I still had my secret. Every night as I undressed, I checked again. Yes, the lump was still there; growing, puckering my skin around it, looking more and more like the cancer it really was. I began to avoid undressing in front of Jasper in case he noticed. I couldn't lie on my right side in bed and cuddle him because it hurt so much. I tried unsuccessfully to swap our sides of the bed, much to his confusion and annoyance.

After I got home from the tour, Jasper asked me if I would please stop trying to work and just be there with him. He felt safe with me at home, he was scared to be alone, and I, of course, immediately agreed. I agreed fully and willingly. I wanted nothing else but to be whatever he needed me to be.

I had organised a surprise trip to see Liverpool football team play at Anfield in August. Jasper was so excited and happy; he loved sport and his team with a passion. It was wonderful to see him animated and upbeat. We went on from Liverpool to Southern Ireland and stayed in a friend's converted barn for a week. It was beautiful, bittersweet and sad. Jasper couldn't walk far; his energy was very low, and a deep depression had begun to bite. As it rained all week, we watched endless episodes of *Breaking Bad*, laughing at the protagonist's story, so like our own in terms of diagnosis. We couldn't have known it would become a recurring theme for us over the next while. Carrots and cannabis oil – who could have known they would become so important?

All summer long I had been suffering almost daily from a cluster of visual migraines that had been plaguing me for months. While on tour I'd had several debilitating episodes a day. I didn't know it at the time, but it is now my belief that this was a direct result of my body flooding with oestrogen.

Finally, in late September 2013, I went to my GP. She took one look at my breast and arranged an appointment at the oncology breast unit for the following week.

I walked slowly back home to tell Jasper. I was shocked, exhausted and still disbelieving. However, I knew it was true; there had been a shadow, a spectre in my life for a long time. I had been in denial for many, many months. I walked back into our flat and he said, half-jokingly, "What's the matter, love? You look even more freaked out than normal."

I confessed to what I had been hiding. Aw, my poor husband; my gorgeous, brave man. My love. I couldn't bear to hurt him. I just couldn't bear to bring more anxiety and worry to him. He couldn't believe I had kept the lump from him for all those months. He was extremely angry with me to begin with, something I had never experienced from him before, and he felt betrayed, as we had never kept anything from each other, never lied even by omission. Eventually, I made him understand; it was all for love. I couldn't bear for him to feel as I had when he was diagnosed. I knew it would tear our fragile world further apart, and so it did. I explained to him that I didn't want the focus to be pulled from him to me and I was so overloaded with worry and grief for him and what we were losing, it felt deeply wrong to throw another bomb like breast cancer into our edge-of-coping lives; we were so broken how could we possibly deal with anymore illness. However, my secret was well and truly out of the box now.

A Time to Grow

Through the winter of 2013 we finally made the very difficult decision to grow our own cannabis. It was the only way we could guarantee we would be using the strains needed for medicinal use. These needed to be high in CBD: cannabidiol is just one of more than eighty-five cannabinoids found in the cannabis plant, and low in THC; tetrahydrocannabinol is the principal psychoactive constituent of cannabis. However, some of the newer research suggested there were better results at a fifty-fifty split of the two, also written as 1:1.

It was also the only way we could begin to afford the treatment. Impossible to buy, even if we could have afforded it at £3,000 per treatment. We began our grow using seeds from the Critical Mass strain, a fifty-fifty split between THC and CBD, and once again we felt hugely empowered and full of hope. Jasper researched a lot himself, using books and forums on the internet; particularly *Marijuana Horticulture: The Indoor/Outdoor Medical Grower's Bible* by Jorge Cervantes, and the growers' website UK420. He became lively again, enjoying his daily tasks of minding, watering, feeding and tending his plants. We grew indoors, under lights, using only organic feed and in organic soil. I was very fearful we would be busted and both end up in jail. I was scared of spending his last months in a maelstrom of police charges, court appearances and jail sentences. He didn't care. He was resolute in his decisions; he was saving his own life, and how could anyone possibly argue with that? We kept our own counsel, telling very few people what we were doing and never posting on Facebook about it.

Our plants grew through the winter of 2013 and spring of 2014, and we collected and dried flower buds, grew more, and collected and dried more. Our stash grew slowly, but never to the huge amounts we needed. We began a second grow at a friend's house, and Jasper continued to take the oil we had previously made.

However, at the same time, I felt him retreating in that spring of 2014. He started to balk at our highly nutritious, mostly vegan/vegetarian diet, saying if he was going to die, he wanted meat pies and biscuits. It was all I could do to keep the juice regime going for both of us. He also clearly needed fats and calories as he was beginning to lose weight. I understood we were diverging in terms of dietary requirements. Jasper was advised by his oncologist to eat lots of cream and ice cream, and to have a diet high in processed foods. I couldn't see a way to keep going with two separate diets, I just didn't have the time, and so my diet largely fell by the wayside to make room for what he needed. I was happy to defer my needs. I wanted whatever kept him well enough and happy.

Reading back through my few, very sporadic diary entries from this period, which were my safe place, it's clear that the diary became my friend, a place to talk freely about my loneliness, my fear and isolation. As such, it received the darkest parts of my journey, and I am distressed by my entries for April 2014.

Diary entry, April 2014

I have been through many cycles of grief and loneliness this past year, and a version of hell, but somehow this week is different. I feel hopeless. I think he is giving up. He is opting for leaving me. I try to support him in his choices, but this one I can't figure. I know I must let him go, but how can I do that? I don't know how. I try to let go a bit, but all that happens is I pull back into myself. Then I want to be alone. At least then I don't have to pretend, I don't have to put on a brave face, but that leaves us with a horrible distance between us. He doesn't understand because he doesn't know that I have figured it out. He gives it away, though, the lack. I find myself asking silently, Who cares for me while I care for you? It seems there are many people paying lip service to support, but how come I can't think of a single person to call at midnight to share my pain? This is too hard.

Of course, there were several people I could have called; the lack was within me. I was too bewildered, too hurt, and too lost to be able to reach out.

Through the early spring of 2014 I found a way of taking some time for me, a way of keeping my sanity. I had spent some time the previous year applying to various charities for money to take us away from our lives, to have respite breaks from our half-life. Our friends and family had also chipped in. I had done well with my applications, and we were very well supported, particularly by the Musicians Benevolent Fund, now called Help Musicians, alongside various other charities. I holed up in a local but out-of-the-way hotel with a swimming pool, for one night just before my next breast operation and reconstruction, and I submerged myself in water as much as I could, trying to wash away my bitterness, my grief. *I am seeking clarity – how do I feel? I am seeking solace – where? I am seeking peace – unattainable. I am seeking a resolution – I cannot bear to live this life, and I cannot bear to live the one to come. But it's all there is, and so I must stay strong, for now.*

We had now grown enough organic bud for Jasper to do a proper treatment. We cooked again, very successfully, and then spent a crazy sixty days through May and June 2014 with him doubling his dose of oil every four days until he was up to the gram a day needed to fight cancer. Those were crazy, strange days. He was utterly wiped out by the dose; unable to function really, and once more I was in sole charge of running the house, shopping, cooking and juicing. Jasper was sleeping loads, and when awake he was vague and isolated, too stoned to function. His memory was completely shot. We would have the same conversations over and over, with him not remembering anything we had said only minutes prior.

We also had times of deep love and care. We snuggled up together on the couch. We fell in love again. We laughed a lot; silly, stoned laughter that was so good for the soul, and at times had us in tears of joy and emotional pain. These were bittersweet times indeed. Make no mistake, reader: cannabis oil is not an easy option for many reasons; the legality and the issues of providing what you need to make a treatment being only a part of it. It's also a hefty dunt to the body and mind; the patient requires constant care and help to function, to eat and prepare meals, and to do the normal daily tasks of life. I think it can be likened to chemotherapy in this respect. Someone taking oil in these massive doses is very toxic and wobbly. We were lucky in that weed was something we had dabbled in, in our previous life. It wasn't too far a jump for us. I can imagine, though, that for someone not versed in being stoned and operating outside the law, the strain may make the whole process intolerable.

My diary entry for 4th May is so hopeful:

Diary, 4th May 2014

Something has changed – I don't know if I can write it. It's intangible. I see it in tiny glimpses that have no expression – maybe it's a knowing, maybe that's it. It translates as:

> *Golden light,*
> *Much laughter,*
> *Lots closer,*
> *Lots of cuddles and warmth,*
> *As if this is the time I will want to remember.*

My diary entry for 8th May is more focused – how I wish I had written in my diary on many more days. I can't believe now, reading back, what we went through. I am amazed to find I have forgotten so much.

Diary, 8th May 2014

Early summer is upon us – bluebells and forget-me-nots in abundance. [Forget-me-nots were always Jasper's favourite – our back garden was a sea of blue at this time of year.] *The new growth is everywhere. I can feel my own sap rising, as it does every year at this time. I feel it in me, the impatience, the need to keep moving, the need to make big, impossible plans, the urge to move forward. I feared this time of year coming around. I wondered how I would cope with our half-life, our inability to make any plans, our fear.*

Jasper is up to one gram of cannabis oil today. He's been on half a gram these past four days, properly stoned and hard to reach sometimes. I worry he is lonely, although he won't admit to being so. I find it hard not to involve him in day-to-day life, just as he finds it hard to rest and stop. What a strange journey we are travelling together. I can't know how it will go. All I see around me are signs that he is thinking it will end. My love, the love of my life, in my heart I want you to try harder to stay here with me, to go that extra distance with your diet, make it count; but I fear you have already decided and you are merely humouring me as we slowly wind down our life together. This is part of my grief alone, and I know I can't keep you here just by my sheer will, and the effort is distracting us from the deep love that says it doesn't matter. I have become an autocrat, a worrier over stuff that is not my concern. Ultimately, I can only look to my own health and the big questions I am asking myself all the damn time, the biggest of which is – what is the point? How can I become an old lady; what's there for me without you? Poverty? Pain? Grandchildren? Who will I become in the years ahead if I survive this dreadful disease and the urge to end it all?

By now it was June 2014. We felt deep in ourselves that it would be our last summer together and we were determined to have a good one. We talked a lot about how things could go/would go. We were always best friends, and somehow, we managed to have impossible conversations, greatly aided by humour and our deep love for one another. We organised a seaside holiday to Harvest Moon in East Lothian with friends in mid-June and invited lots of folks. The day before we were due to go, and only two days after finishing four weeks of gruelling radiotherapy, I fell badly and managed to break four ribs on my 'good' side. My, oh my – I was utterly miserable and very sore indeed. The holiday went ahead as planned and Jasper had a really good time. Golfing on the beach with Dave, late night bonfires, lots of laughter with our friends, and we even managed to go skinny-dipping one day. He had the time with our pals we wanted him to have, precious time that no one will forget, but for me it was a terribly lonely time. I was utterly broken in heart, spirit and body; grieving, breast cancer, radiotherapy, and now four broken ribs.

Radiotherapy is evil. The doctors tell you it has little or no side effects. I disagree, and understanding a bit more about the process, I can't help but think it will always hurt. The tissues within the blast site contract; they die quickly, instantly, and this causes muscle spasms and rigors. I also suffered hourly bouts of paralysing hot flushes as my kidneys tried in vain to flush out the radioactive toxins. The sunburn was not too bad, though. When Jasper was irradiated, the following winter for spinal tumours, he had an excruciating few days as the tumours reacted and flared. I was astonished and perturbed to see, a few weeks after his radiotherapy, that his belly was bald in the shape of a large rectangle where the radiotherapy beam had passed through his back to his stomach and out the other side. This was chilling to see.

I consider driving myself, alone, to radiotherapy for five days a week, for over four weeks, and lying down in the beam while the technicians scurried from the room as the alarm went off, a barrier dropped across the doorway and the beam hit, to be one of the bravest things I have done. I can't begin to tell you how terrified it made me, and how wrong I felt it to be; how fundamentally wrong. I am a child of the '60s; radiation was the bogeyman. It is a sci-fi terror that has stayed with me.

Facebook post, 1st June 2014

One of the associated difficulties of living with long-term illness is the patience required by friends and family to keep being able and willing to support us through the peaks and troughs. For all of this I am so grateful. xxx

Facebook post, 13th June 2014

Finally. The end of nineteen days of radiotherapy today. The medics tell me the effects continue to develop for another two weeks and then it will be September earliest before I begin to feel well. Ho-hum. For the curious: yes, it is utterly gruelling and exhausting, and yes, it does hurt, sometimes very much. This is due to all the surgical intervention I have had, apparently, and is not the same for everyone. Anyway, the point of this post is, I DID IT. It's done. Onward… into summer, weddings, the island, holidays, Towersey Folk Festival, sunshine, good times, maybe even some (blame it on the) boogie. Happy Friday 13th, folks, hope it's a good one. We think it will be an auspicious day. Bring it on. xx

Facebook post, 16th July 2014

Turns out I am allergic to some of the dissolving stitches. Just had another two 'stitch abscesses' removed; that makes six in all so far in the past week. My surgeon thinks this may be the reason I didn't heal after my first round of breast cancer surgery way back in October 2013, and the basis for the months and months of infection… There's lots of these stitches in me, so I "just have to wait for my body to push them out and the hospital to remove them". NICE. You may wonder why I am telling you this… It's because lots of lovely folks keep messaging me asking how I am. People are mind-blowingly lovely and amazing and generous. THANK YOU, PEOPLES!!! x

Facebook post, 22nd July 2014

This has truly been the craziest and most profound past two years. Living with not one but two cancer diagnoses in the house is challenging, to say the least. There have been sad times and hard times, happy times and glad times, and lots of times when just somehow getting through the day is all there is. The past two or three months have been particularly tough and lonely, and it's been impossible to post much publicly about how we really are. The love and support we receive is monumental and at times quite overwhelming. This is one of those times for me. THANK YOU, FRIENDS and THANK YOU, FAMILY – thank you FOR YOUR LOVE. xx

Marino Branch
Brainse Marino
Tel: 8336297

Cannabis Oil

Since Jasper's diagnosis in January 2013, ten months previously, I had been researching cannabis oil as a treatment and a cure for cancer. The information was out there and readily available; it was all over the superhighway. As a cure for cancer cannabis oil was becoming well documented by people working out-with the normal medical models. We had looked at different ways of obtaining the huge amounts of cannabis needed; we researched the new science and had even, for a brief time, considered moving to America. However, we quickly realised we could not absent ourselves from family and friends for months on end, on another continent, when time was so short, and decided it wasn't possible for us to go down the cannabis oil treatment route. The amounts of bud needed were just staggering: sixteen ounces of weed makes sixty grams of oil, which equals one treatment, and the whole scenario seemed impossible to achieve. My diagnosis changed that thinking. I decided I wanted to treat with oil, and so we agreed to attempt a cook. Three days before I was due in for my breast surgery found us at a friend's empty house, in the garden, with four ounces of street weed, a step-by-step guide from the internet, a load of 99% proof alcohol (isopropyl), a rice cooker, some plastic syringes and a gung-ho attitude. Note: this would be impossible today (2019) due to increased restrictions on buying highly flammable materials, because of the high level of terror threat in the UK and beyond.

We made our first batch of oil in late October 2013 and were surprised at how easy the process was. We felt empowered and in charge of our own destiny. This is a vital part of the healing process in this type of treatment. However, we also managed to overdose ourselves horribly. The amounts for consumption are so tiny; beware, dear reader, and be very careful. The starting dose equivalent to half a grain of rice per day is a huge amount for the body to take. We had way too much and both became very tripped out and unwell – made much worse by the fact we were using street weed, grown with a high THC content for the intoxicating effects, and not the high CBD bud we would later grow ourselves. I remember lying on the couch at home, not knowing who I was, where I was or what was outside the room! I was fortunate to have experienced a 'trip' in my younger days, and common sense got me through the terrifying disconnection I experienced that first time. I knew nothing apart from it would end at some point, and I would come back to myself. It's important also to note here that there are other side effects from cannabis oil: it drops blood pressure and so can make you quite dizzy, and it's a stomach irritant and therefore should always be taken with food, from a syringe on a small piece of bread. We also discovered it made us very giggly and we would hear each other in separate parts of the flat chuckling to ourselves. It felt so good to laugh and to feel light. We would regularly set each other off laughing from a different room, and then immediately come find one another just to giggle and cuddle.

We decided Jasper's need for oil was greater than mine. We had only made a few grams of oil, nowhere near the sixty grams needed for one treatment, i.e. one gram a day for sixty days, but incredibly, a tiny daily dose was enough to change his outlook. His depression lifted. He slept deeply, and his appetite and his colour returned, along with his humour. We felt positive for the first time in over a year. This was good medicine, if only in terms of a palliative. We decided we needed to find enough to treat us both. Somehow.

N.B. I am aware I have previously skipped over my breast cancer diagnosis. The following Facebook posts take us back to 2013, and the following pages help to clarify what breast cancer meant for our family.

Facebook post, 10th November 2013

Hi, pals; so… you may have noticed, it's a cancer epidemic out there. Jasper and I have some news which perhaps you have heard already; if not we hope you don't mind hearing it here. It's all gone a bit bonkers.

I have very recently been diagnosed with breast cancer. It's a Grade 1 tumour (which is the best grade to have), it's operable and my prognosis is excellent. We should have the full picture of spread (if any) etc. by the middle of December. My operation is booked for 19th November, then two to three weeks' recovery, chemotherapy and radiotherapy through January/February, then tamoxifen for a while, alongside natural remedies.

Obviously, considering Jasper's diagnosis of Stage 4 lung cancer in January, this is just barmy and unbelievable. Maybe we will wake up soon.

We are shocked and things are happening at such a fast pace it's very difficult to keep up. We are already exhausted trying to adjust to Jasper's prognosis and managing his day-to-day health, and so this is hard to accommodate.

People are asking; what they can do? Please send healing love, you lovely loves (we are fully stocked with carrots). Please keep asking what can be done; we seldom know the answer, but it's lovely to be asked. Eat more carrots. Come around, make a juice, wash the juicer. Ladies, look to your boobs! Gents, look to your ladies' boobs... and your own bits too. Please, although really appreciated, don't PM me the very many cures for cancer as I just don't have the time or energy to check them out. I have been researching natural cures throughout 2013 for Jasper, and we have both decided on our approaches and feel they are the right ones for us, for now anyway.

Please share this if you want to; giving bad news is so hard. I feel it's better to get it out there ASAP and then we can all look to whatever comes next.

Erm, so, life's a bugger, hey; what are the chances? WTF, lightning strikes, best foot forward, chin up, keep smiling, keep laughing, keep keeping on... and all that stuff. Are we in a series of Lost?

Thanks for all the 'holding tight' support we have had through the craziness of my diagnosis over the last couple of weeks, and for the past eleven months too.

Lots of love, best wishes and GOOD HEALTH to you. xxxxxxxxxxx

Within two weeks I had a 'large local incision' operation to remove the tumour in my right breast, and I also had several lymph nodes cleared from my right armpit. On 19th November 2013 I was told my cancer was Stage 2a. It had spread to lymph nodes in my armpit and was oestrogen receptive. I should have been in hospital to have it removed months ago. My surgeon reckoned it had been growing in me for twelve to eighteen months, and it was 1.4 centimetres long. I had known, on some level, that it was there; it had been calling to me in my dreams, yelling at me through my intense visual migraines and mocking me in mirrors. It had been demanding I wake up and pay attention, testing my desire for death and my will to live, to outlive my husband. It's a sick joke, to be fair, and some days we laughed out loud at the ludicrousness of our situation; yes indeed, we laughed a lot. We laughed long and hard. Our humour grew darker, and we held on tighter.

I honestly can't say how long I suspected I had cancer; I ignored the signs leading up to the definite moment of recognition, which came in July while on tour. A B&B mirror told me I could no longer pretend it wasn't happening. Although I still managed to hide it for another two whole months; how, I have no idea. The stress I was under with Jasper's prognosis and, I firmly believe, the cancer, as mentioned previously, was giving me clusters of visual migraines that affected me almost daily all through that very lonely summer of 2013. However, I haven't had a single migraine since my tumour was removed.

Facebook post, 20th November 2013

*YAH! Home, sore, tired, wobbly, blue, fine. Typing is hard.
I'm just about to hide away for the day and rest up, but
really wanted to say thanks so much, folks; all those lovely
messages really kept me going yesterday. You ROCK.*

*Amazing care from Ward 6 and the cancer team in
Edinburgh. Thank you!*

*Rani and Jasper, a fine breakout last night to get
me home. Even though I was yellow, dizzy and shaky (I
managed to fool the ward staff but not you two, hey!)
and I was not really fit for home… you got me home, and
today is so much better for it. xx*

*Love, love, love to you all and your wonderful
messages. xxxxxxxxxxxx*

All around us professional people were deciding what treatment,
what drugs and what outcomes. We were completely at sea. I
had foolishly demanded to get straight home on the night of my
operation, so concerned was I to be home, in my place as wife,
with Jasper's care more important than mine. I woke that night at
2am, in my own bed, feeling as though a huge weight had landed
on my chest. In fact, I had had a massive bleed, a haematoma,
which had pooled in the lower part of my breast, below my
wound. I was unaware of this, and the impending infection that
was brewing. I woke one night soon after, confused as to why I felt
sticky, to find our bed covered in blood.

December saw me admitted to hospital again for five days on
IV antibiotics. I was terrified I might spend our last Christmas
together in the cancer ward, but thankfully I was released again
on 22nd December. The haematoma was identified, and then

began a five-month-long nightmare of infections, hospital admissions, more surgeries, and antibiotics. I had to undergo gruesome dressing changes, where my deep and infected wound was packed with inches of soft colloidal gauze. My wound was packed by the consultant, my daughter, the GP, and by the district nurses. It was also packed, tentatively but willingly, for ten days by my courageous husband when we ran away to the Canary Islands in January 2014 for some much-needed sunshine. We went against all medical advice. We laughed and joked together over this ritual: "How deep is your love?", "In sickness and in more sickness", and "Hey, how broken are we?" We felt so free, despite our many limitations. It was very good for our souls to say, "To hell with it, we are getting on the plane."

Immediately on our return from the Canaries (the very next day in fact), we began a nightmare two weeks. I was hospitalised and had another general anaesthetic. The infection was scraped from my breast tissue and I was attached, by the wound on my breast, to a sucking machine to try and pull the poison from my tissues. All the time I'm thinking, *We are wasting our precious time, the months are ticking by. I must be well; we have so little time.*

Over the years we beat a path between our house and the cancer centre, sometimes three or four days a week, every week, between Jasper's care and mine, plus our regular mental-health-saving visits to Maggie's Centre.

Facebook post, 4th February 2014

Hello again,
What a crazy couple of weeks it's been since we got home from our holidays. I have been attached to a

machine since my op two weeks ago and I have been in hiding; thanks for the texts and calls. Hoping the machine is going to be detached tomorrow and I can finally get on with getting well; it's nearly twelve weeks since my initial op, and the game's wearing very thin.

Many thanks indeed to the folks who dropped by over the past two weeks and made a juice or two, or brought us food. xxx

Cooking Oil and Stitches

In early February 2014 I had my 'machine' removed and many internal and external stitches put into my breast. The very next day we were due to go to a friend's house to make more oil. Cannabis oil can only be cooked outside; the fumes from the isopropyl are so toxic and explosive. I remember that it was raining slightly, so I stood for ages as the isopropyl reduced and the oil was made, holding a large golf umbrella, shielding the oil from the rain as we cooked. By the time we got back in the car to drive home, I was in agony. Something had happened deep in my breast. I lay on the couch at home, quite unable to breathe and in inexplicable pain. I was utterly terrified, knowing I would have to return to the breast clinic the next day to be investigated. Jasper paced the house all night, deeply worried about me and repeatedly telling me he had never seen me look so unwell.

The next day I had my external stitches removed and, to my surgeon's horror and my own, he discovered all the internal stitches were busted open and needed to be redone. The tissue in my breast was horribly strained, fragile from months of surgeries and infection. I told him I had done it hanging up the washing. He was sorely unimpressed with me.

I had refused six months of chemotherapy, I had refused ten years of tamoxifen, and I had also refused four weeks of radiotherapy. I just couldn't face the added disruption to our already shattered lives. Maybe I simply liked the idea of dying, too. Radiotherapy, chemotherapy and tamoxifen were, to me, a litany of wrongness. I fretted so hard over these decisions; I woke every morning in a sweat of fear that I really didn't know what was best for my body. But through that fear there was the feeling, *I am aware there is a different choice – choosing life, for now, to spend with my husband, being relatively well, travelling, loving, laughing, living, choosing death before old age.*

It's not that I didn't want treatment, but the treatment I wanted and had researched at great length was illegal: cannabis oil. It is still illegal in the UK, but since I started my research in early 2013, its use has spread across the USA as a legal and viable way to treat cancer and other diseases. Spain is also way ahead, and other countries are catching up.

At this point I decided to really go hard with our diet. I gave up all dairy after reading Jane Plant's book *Your Life in Your Hands: Understand, Prevent and Overcome Breast Cancer and Ovarian Cancer.* I increased the vegan aspect, cut out even more sugar, and upped the oxygenating foods in our diet. Jasper was not impressed but I bullied him into it, for a while anyway.

Jasper was still doing OK with his health; the Tarceva side effects had settled a bit and the drug was holding the tumours steady. By April 2014 I was free of infection. I was very lucky indeed to be called in to see the head of the breast unit, a maverick surgeon, Professor Dixon, who, having read my recent email to him, wondering what he thought about cannabis oil as a treatment, had decided I needed a good talking-to for refusing the conventional treatments offered. The professor took one look at my battered, scarred, shrunken and misshapen right breast and told me I was still a young woman (forty-seven), with my whole life ahead of me and he wanted to go back in and reconstruct me. Not just my broken breast, but my left one too, to make them good, to make them even. I realised, when I burst into tears in his office at this prospect, how depressed I was about my body image, how much I needed to be 'fixed'. I agreed to the reconstruction. Thank God I did as the next operation found another tumour in my scar tissue which had been missed in the original operation back in November. I then agreed to the radiotherapy and promised him I would take tamoxifen (which I didn't). More time 'wasted'.

Facebook post, May 2014

Hiya, pals, hope you're all fine. We have been living very quietly here; I have been healing and mending, and Jasper is doing well. Thanks for the messages, and special thanks also for the super-strong support from parents and pals; we really couldn't have managed without you. I have been able to rest much more and heal much better.

A wee update for those who are interested. The pathology on the scar tissue taken away in my recent round of reconstructive surgery in mid April showed another tumour. I am reeling a bit; we could really catch a break here… and I have another infection. Hey-ho, back on the antibiotics.

I'm at a radiotherapy measure-up session today, so will get my dates for the next stint. (Update: radiotherapy dates are five days a week, 19th May to 13th June.) Then me and him can get on with summer.

I'm enjoying spending time away from Facebook and find I am back to writing on real paper, composing weird prose, and also enjoying sending letters. Feeling the need for physical, not so much virtual. Sending out much love and thanks indeed. xxxxxxxx

Very generalised good practices for an anti-cancer diet

I researched the following strands of dietary health over several years, and I also took lots of advice from my craniosacral therapist Susana. The info is very general, and I would say that talking to a nutritionist or kinesiologist about a particular cancer and approach is never a bad idea as the following may not be suitable for everyone.

- To be successful with your diet for 80–90% of the time is generally thought to be extremely worthwhile in terms of health, and also in terms of actually sticking to it long term. The regime can become tedious and you may feel you are 'missing out' if you don't give yourself a break now and again. That could be every day, or a day a week, or a fortnight, where you just have whatever you fancy.
- In basic terms you are aiming for a diet high in alkalising foods and low in acidic foods. Cancer cannot thrive in an alkaline environment. Our modern diets are incredibly acidic and a breeding ground for tumours and other illnesses.
- A cancer-fighting diet is very high in dark, leafy green vegetables, and high in whole grains and

'good' fats like avocados. This diet requires lemons (they are alkalising), cold-pressed olive oils, coconut oil and flax oil. The diet is mostly organic, mostly vegan, very low in both natural and processed sugars, and low in refined fats. Avoid all things white – potatoes, white bread, white rice, white spaghetti; these are all acidic.

- The organic element is hugely important, particularly regarding juicing and also with meat consumption. I aim for a 90% organic approach. This is something I am very fussy about as I believe cancer is caused, in part, by the pesticides, toxins and dioxins in our food and the packaging that surrounds it. Plastic is the enemy in my house. I have a stainless-steel washing-up bowl and, as much as possible, I avoid storing food in plastic containers.

- Water is good! And it helps prevent acidity. Aim to drink at least four pints of filtered water per day. This is what your body needs just to be still. Avoid bottled water and sparkling water; both are very acidic and bottled water, left in sunlight or refilled from the tap, is a definite no-no as the dioxins in the plastic leak out. These dioxins are implicated in the huge rise in breast cancers worldwide.

- Alcohol is very high in sugar and is also very acidic. Try to buy organic alcohol as it tends to not have sulphates added, which cause some of the harm.

- I found decreasing my sugar intake really helped me with sugar cravings, and the same was true of bread. I swapped sugar for a small amount of honey. Sugar feeds tumours, so avoid where possible.

- I eat very little processed food. I juice four times

a day (on a good day!) and try to drink water about twenty minutes before a meal. Don't drink too much water with a meal as it cools the food and creates sludge in your stomach that's hard to digest.

- I became 90% vegan for a while after reading Jane Plant's book *Your Life in Your Hands* – a weighty, scientific tome that was difficult to read but gave me a very clear idea of just why milk and cancers, particularly breast cancer, go hand in hand. However, although attempting to give up all dairy and to eat vegan, I will eat cheese if I'm eating out and I enjoy a good steak occasionally. I also still eat eggs, and sometimes fish or chicken. It is worth bearing in mind that, cheese is, generally acidic.

- I have taken some elements of Gerson therapy and applied them to my lifestyle. The Gerson diet can cure cancer very successfully, but it requires proper support for the whole of your system, as it can become incredibly toxic to the liver. Toxicity can be recognised as feeling sick, headachy, and/or suffering sweats, irritability and joint pain. If juicing in large amounts every day, it's advisable to self-administer coffee enemas. These are easy to perform and have an amazing boost value to the liver. See http://gerson.org for more info on how to manage aspects of this diet. Buy only organic green coffee and use only filtered water for enemas. http://gerson.org/pdfs/How_Coffee_Enemas_Work.pdf

- Juicing: use only a masticating juicer, or 'slow' juicer, as oppose to a centrifugal juicer. The juicer is your friend; research what you need and aim to spend a decent amount of money. My juicers have included a Samson and a JR, both costing upwards of £200, but I use them every day and feel they are worth their weight in gold. Only juice organic, always wash fruit and vegetables thoroughly, and drink the juice as soon as it is made as the enzymes break down very quickly after being 'processed'. Don't buy ready-made juices; they have very little nutritional value. For juicers see http://www. juicyretreats.com/#!jr-ultra-juicers/c1nv4 and http://www.samsonjuicers.com/

- Golden paste – turmeric powder, black pepper and coconut oil – is a daily staple for me. Two small teaspoons per day, taken morning and night. Always take with food and build up the dose slowly. Golden paste is anti-cancer, anti-inflammatory, and an extremely effective antidepressant. Don't buy ready-made pills or potions; they are nowhere near as effective as what you make yourself. It's extremely simple to make your own and store it in the freezer in weekly batches. For general information on effects (and side effects) see http://www.turmericforhealth. com/faqs/comprehensive-list-of-turmeric-faqs.

Here's a typical day. This is a very good day, and not every day is this good! Starting early is essential for me, to fit it all in. I won't state 'organic' on everything, but organic is definitely the preferred option.

- On waking, a glass of filtered water with fresh lemon juice.
- Cup of tea with a small amount of honey (white tea is better as it contains less caffeine).
- Breakfast: porridge, made with either water or almond milk, chia seeds, two Brazil nuts, prunes, dried cranberries, sunflower seeds, and fresh fruit. Half a teaspoon of golden paste on the side.
- Carrot, apple and ginger juice: 350 grams of carrots, half an apple, an inch of ginger and a teaspoon of flax oil. (Scrub carrots and apple well, and peel ginger – no need to peel organic carrots.)
- Small glass of water twenty minutes before lunch.
- Green juice: a handful of kale, a small beetroot, a portion of sweet potato, a stick of celery, quarter of a cucumber, a small handful of fresh wheatgrass (grow your own; it's easy), half a lemon (peeled, but keep the white pith) and a teaspoon of cider vinegar (alkalising).
- Lunch: whole-wheat spaghetti with salad, or homemade pumpkin/squash and butter bean soup, or hummus and oatcakes.
- Small glass of water.
- Citrus juice: two oranges and the other half of the lemon.
- Dinner: steamed fish; oily fish is best, but I prefer haddock or cod (make sure haddock is not dyed using colourings), or puy lentil stew with sweet potatoes, or lentil curry. Add a good handful of leafy greens, the darker the better, plus green beans, broccoli and carrots.
- Carrot, apple and ginger juice, as above.
- A glass of water.

In March 2017 I began the Whole30 programme https:// whole30.com/whole30-program-rules/ – I'm on day twenty-six as I write. It's a food elimination diet and it cuts out wheat, dairy, sugar, cereals, grains, beans, pulses and legumes for thirty days. I've been eating meat, eggs, vegetables, fish and fruit, and feel well on it.

The Fantasist, the Hopefuls and the Black, Black Oil

Late July 2014 and we are following a lead from an old pal who reckons he has found a doctor in England who can help us with treating Jasper's cancer with cannabis oil. This friend has heard on the grapevine that we're attempting to collate the very large amounts needed for each treatment – sixty grams of oil, over sixty days, is considered one treatment. Several treatments may be needed to treat cancer.

The process basically involves making essential oil out of cannabis flowers (bud), and requires approximately sixteen ounces of cannabis per treatment. A hugely expensive undertaking at roughly £3,500 (street value) per treatment – if you were to buy it, and even then you wouldn't be getting the right strain of plant; you need something very high in CBD as opposed to THC. CBD is the active ingredient in medical marijuana; THC is the component of the plant that gets you high. Fifty-fifty or 1:1 is considered to be a good mix. As I mentioned previously, we had done a huge amount of research. Below is a quote which explains how it is effective and why we can use it.

There are over 400 natural compounds in medical marijuana and, of these, eighty are only found in cannabis plants. These eighty special compounds are known as cannabinoids. Cannabinoids relieve symptoms of illness by attaching to receptors in the brain that look for similar compounds that occur in the human body, such as dopamine.

There are five major cannabinoids in medical marijuana that are particularly effective for relieving symptoms of illness, and each one produces different physical and psychological effects. This is why certain strains of medical marijuana are bred to have different amounts of each cannabinoid and are recommended for different conditions. http://www.unitedpatientsgroup.com/resources/how-medical-marijuana-works

As the above quote shows, there are many active ingredients in medical marijuana, and I recommend researching thoroughly for what strain suits a particular cancer.

When we began researching this in 2013 the science was in its infancy in the UK. However, many states in America and Spain were leading the field in research and legal usage, and it was easy for me to research the use of cannabis oil as a treatment for cancer. I am particularly indebted to the Canadian Rick Simpson for his contribution to the cause. Simpson was the first person to treat skin cancer – his own – with cannabis oil. He then supplied many people for years and documented many recoveries from cancer, using oil. He was prosecuted several times by the Canadian authorities and has lived in exile in Europe. Rick Simpson has paid a heavy price for his willingness to help others, all for no fee or personal gain. I believe that what he intuited has become a much more exact science, and it's possible to grow and treat far more effectively than in the past. I also found invaluable advice and research through Jeff Ditchfield's work here in the UK, along with his work on *Project Storm*, and also from Professor Manuel Guzmán at the Department of Biochemistry and Molecular Biology at the Complutense University of Madrid.

[Guzmán's] PhD and post-doctoral research focused on the study of the regulation of liver and brain lipid metabolism. Since 2001 he has been involved in the study of how the active components of cannabis (cannabinoids) act in the body, with special emphasis on the molecular mechanisms of action and on understanding how cannabinoids control cell generation and death.

https://www.jeffditchfield.com/professor-manuel-guzman/

As I write this part in January 2016, the UK position has come on leaps and bounds, to the point that, as I walked down Sauchiehall Street in Glasgow recently, I came across a 'police box business' selling CBD oils in various strains and grades. When I asked the bloke tending the shop if it was legal, he proudly told me he was the first business in Scotland to be granted a Home Office licence to produce and provide medicinal cannabis oils. However, it is only legal as it contains no THC and research has suggested that both compounds (THC and CBD) work holistically; they are, in fact, greater than the sum of their parts. If only Jasper and I had had access to this type of medicine three years ago when we began this particular aspect of our journey, who knows what difference it might have made. Three years ago we considered moving to America to access the type of medicine I can now legally buy here.

Even with the two grows going consecutively, we were still struggling to provide what we needed for ourselves. It was hard enough to obtain enough for one cancer, never mind two. We telephoned the doctor in England who had been recommended by our old friend and asked for a meeting. He invited us to his place, and we made the arrangements to travel south. By this point in August 2014, Jasper was really struggling with his health; he was exceptionally tired, the cancer had spread further into his bones (previously it had just been in his ribs, but we now suspected his shoulder blade or clavicle was compromised and possibly his spine) and he was finding life very depressing, painful and difficult. We were invited to attend a friend's festival as their guests of honour, where Jasper would introduce his old company to the crowd, on a night dedicated to their work over the years. We would camp amongst old friends and try and be 'in the world'. We borrowed a friend's camper van and set off. As mentioned previously I was just past my four weeks of radiotherapy, as well as another operation in which another tumour had been found, and I was nursing four broken ribs after a nasty fall. We weren't in great shape, but we were hopeful that we could finally access the huge amounts needed to help us.

Dr John was a strange man, and I was immediately very unsure of him. He avoided my questions about what strains of plant he would recommend or what strains he was using to treat his 'patients'. He was also a bit short on information about his research and his other patients. He told us he was currently treating twenty cancer patients, all under the radar, not sanctioned by any medical body and all for the good of underground medical science; no fees were ever applied. He also told us he had previously (circa 2007) been given a research grant by an English university to grow medical marijuana and to treat seven people to the end of their life. I asked him how many had survived; he answered one. I was particularly dismayed when he informed Jasper that, as he had Stage 4 lung cancer, he was going to die, so why not just have some fun? To me this was callous, and I felt he just didn't have the kind of manner, or manners, a person would have if they lived and worked amongst the terminally ill.

We left Dr John's place with Jasper in high spirits. I jokingly kept saying, and continued to do so, that Dr John was a fantasist of the highest order and I didn't believe in him. Jasper, as always, believed the best of anyone and couldn't conceive of why someone would make it all up.

We arrived home in late August, exhausted and not knowing, but intuiting, that Jasper was heading into the last six months of his life. Very quickly our old pal, who had set up the meeting with Dr John, began to send large amounts of oil through the post, and Jasper began another 'sixty grams in sixty days' treatment. However, the first batch he sent we returned, as it clearly still contained isopropyl. This was evident by the burn in our throats and the smell, which once you have completed your own cook, you can identify easily as isopropyl. I was worried about what were we taking. It felt very scary; we weren't in control of what we were imbibing, and because it arrived by post and we went to the post office to sign for it, the process felt very unreliable, and possibly, could lead to a visit from the police.

Fast-forward to January 2016. I had a phone call last week from a friend to say that I had been correct in what my gut instinct told me. Dr John was indeed a fantasist. He had been busted in May 2015 with 150 plants and no other patients. Jasper was the only patient, and, it turns out, Dr John was not a doctor, he never received any research grants, he never grew plants to treat patients, he grew plants to make money, and we had been a cover story for him.

All this is, in itself, horribly upsetting. However, worse was to come. He had named me to his defence lawyers in an attempt to have his upcoming sentence reduced and was searching for me through Facebook and the wider internet. He was trolling the internet and asking people, in places I frequented, how I could be contacted, so I could testify in court that he had supplied us with oil. I immediately removed my own treatment stash from the house and bought a pay-as-you-go 'second cell phone' so I could discuss my position from a place of relative safety without compromising myself. (Yes, the *Breaking Bad* element is an ongoing trope in our story.) I deactivated my Facebook page, Jasper's Facebook page, and also put my website into 'maintenance mode'. This was particularly problematic for me as I was just beginning to be 'back in the world' and was dreading the approach of Jasper's first anniversary. I needed to be in the world. I needed to have contact and support through Facebook.

My friend told me Dr John (not a doctor) is considered to be unstable. He is threatening people, and no one really knows what he may do. Until he is sentenced, I now have to keep my head down. I am, at present, fairly philosophical. I have done nothing wrong. I acted in best faith based on the information given to me. I tried to help my dying husband fulfil his wish to live and to be well. However, this is another one of those lessons. Trust your instinct; it's probably right.

Panics and Hospice

Facebook post, 11th September 2014

Fifteen years ago today I sat in a big field near Edinburgh by myself and wondered:

Would 250 people be able to sit down to dinner in the big top the next day?

Would the weather hold? (It did, it was like today.)

Was I crazy, after years of being certain it's not for me, marrying my lodger,

some juggling dude from away down there?

Turns out all three worked out just fine. Love you, mister. Xx

Facebook post, 14th September 2014, our fifteenth wedding anniversary party

OMG! That was just amazing, what a good do. What a load of love in the room! So many folks, from all over the world, and all through the years. WOW. So much effort put in by folks to make it happen and then to clean it all up again. Amazing soups and cakes, and a whole night of fab music too. Bit shell-shocked to be honest.

In September 2014, a couple of days after our anniversary party and halfway through a respite break at our favourite holiday place, Harvest Moon on the coast, with a small group of close friends, Jasper was hospitalised with a common skin infection, cellulitis. It was during this admission that we decided from now on he would only be admitted to hospice for any pain problems. The hospital was so grim and uncaring. He was not well cared for there and it broke my heart to see it. During that autumn his scans also showed the cancer had found a way around the Tarceva; it was spreading and was now in his spine, his pelvis and one of his adrenal glands. The oncologist was concerned he could lose the use of his legs, become incontinent, and maybe it would spread to his brain. These were terrifying prospects for him and for me too.

Facebook post, 28th September 2014

Hi, it's been a wee while since I did one of these updates; I hope you don't mind receiving it. Things have been pretty bonkers the past two weeks, with Jasper ending up in hospital on IV antibiotics with cellulitis (a very painful skin infection). He is now home and the infection is receding.

Unfortunately, his recent bone scan has shown new tumours in his spine, his clavicle; previously we had suspected spread to his shoulder, and it has also spread to his pelvis. We are both doing OK, with lots of support from family and friends, and yesterday from the Marie Curie nurse, who is amazing and has lifted a huge weight of responsibility of care off my shoulders. She has our back. What a service! She is confident that Jasper will bounce back from the infection and that they can manage his symptoms very well from home, so no need to go back to the hellhole that is the oncology wards. Indescribable.

Thanks so much for all the gifts and cards for our wedding anniversary party. It's been such a roller coaster of emotion and effort this past two weeks, and we are only really beginning to read our cards properly, and ooh and aah over pressies. You guys are mighty! We are truly blessed to have such pals. xx

We contacted our GP and she arranged for a community nurse from Marie Curie to visit us at home and to take over Jasper's medication, apart from the Tarceva. She duly arrived and explained that a place in hospice is not guaranteed but is much more likely if you are already on the hospice's 'books'. She was sure she could help us with some of the symptoms Jasper was experiencing, and that we should be able to access hospice as and when we needed it, providing there was a bed available.

Facebook post, 23rd October 2014

A shedload of pal love, a bit of upping 'n' downing, some wise counsels, a few dates in the diary; me and J have left the waiting room… see you soon. xx

I don't know when they started, the first time. But as autumn came in, Jasper started to experience extreme sweats, panic, shakes and terrors. They would come on every day, beginning at around 4pm, as twilight drew in. He would become claustrophobic, agitated, and unable to sit still. I would find him clawing at his arms and legs, saying he felt as though there were creatures living under his skin that were trying to get out. He would sweat so badly we would be constantly mopping with towels. He became terrified to be alone at all, even in the living room, while I was in the kitchen preparing juices.

I was pretty much room and housebound, or bound to him, if we went for a stroll round the block, which could often calm things down for a bit. These attacks increased in frequency all through winter and into early spring; some nights they would roll, one after another, almost seamless in their joins. I was very frightened and unable to do anything other than be there, hold him while he cried himself out, change and wash his clothes, bedding and towels, and try to distract and comfort him. But it was impossible.

There were nights when, in desperation, I would ring for an on-call doctor; always a lottery as it wouldn't be our GP but someone sent from a central call centre. Our large and airy flat would shrink to tiny during those visits, creating a deeper atmosphere of claustrophobia; Jasper in an agony of soul and spirit, his body expressing all it could through panic. These doctors did not know him, had never met him before, and had only the briefest of notes about his medical records and his medications. They didn't understand this was not him, the terrified small boy he would become during these attacks. Often, they would shrug and say, "It's just a panic attack", not realising this was all evening, every evening, deep into the night and sometimes through the day too. I constantly had to correct their knowledge of what medication he was on and where his cancer had progressed to. Generally, they would give him diazepam to calm him; it rarely worked. He was also taking lorazepam regularly to try and abate panic, which of course furthered the payload of medication on his exhausted body.

There was talk, after a scan, of a shadow on his adrenal gland. I leapt at this information, seeing it as a physical reason for all the symptoms of the attacks. But his oncologist shrugged it off, saying it would be having no effect on his actual health; something I struggled to believe, and still do. As performers our adrenal glands were very used to putting us into fight-or-flight mode. This is a natural response the body has to any stress, and preparing for, performing, and the long comedown afterwards was something we experienced at every gig, to some level.

Medication overload was another real factor. All of the '–pams' – diazepam, lorazepam, temazepam – have a significant effect on the nervous system if taken very regularly, causing anxiety in withdrawal; conversely, the very thing they are supposed to treat.

Jasper had also been taking very large doses of an anti-emetic called metoclopramide; again, this is a drug normally used short term. He had been taking it in ever-increasing doses pretty much since he began the Tarceva medication eighteen months previously. And of course, there was the oil. He had stopped taking this in early autumn 2014. He couldn't deal with the extra load on his body and mind and became convinced it was the cause of the attacks. I remember taking him to Maggie's Centre and the horror on our counsellors' faces as I literally dragged him into the centre, one step at a time; he was almost unconscious, he was so deep within himself. Andy, the centre head, was brilliant; he cleared a room for him and sat for an hour, trying to figure out how to help him. We talked about the metoclopramide and Andy explained Jasper's mental state was probably a reaction to the long-term meds. He immediately phoned the hospice, requesting an urgent review of medication and a consult with the psych doctor. However, as was often the case through this period, there was no consensus from the medical team about this aspect and we never did see the psych doctor.

I think the panic attacks were the hardest to bear, for us both. It was utterly exhausting to be in this cycle, and Jasper became increasingly claustrophobic, withdrawn and depressed. His pain was also increasing, and we ended up going into hospice many times over that last winter. Ironically, the 'admitting' rooms at the hospice were tiny. The place was always full; the two smallest rooms were used when a patient first arrived and they would spend twenty-four to forty-eight hours, or a week if no one moved out of a bigger room, being assessed for medication needs. It was hell for him. The room had one tiny window, a tiny bathroom and enough room for a plastic chair by the bed if you sat sideways. All the staff hated these rooms and said that as soon as they could build another wing on the hospice, they would become store cupboards.

I shamelessly walked the corridors, looking for signs that a room might become vacant soon. People came and went, back home or not. The sign on a door that said, *Do not enter without first speaking to a member of staff* meant someone was dying. I badgered staff to have Jasper moved to a larger room. I couldn't stop trying to do the best for him. It drove Jasper crazy. He hated me making a fuss, but expected me to be there at all hours, sitting sideways on a plastic chair, coaxing him through another attack. We would argue about it. The nurses would come in and ask him if he was sore, and he would smile and say no, frustrating the hell out of me, as I knew how much pain he was in and the reason we were in there was to get his level of medication up so he could go home. Round and round we would go. I resented him very much at this time for making me work all the harder, and all so that he didn't seem to be making a fuss.

November 28th 2014 is my next diary entry – I think that a lot of the time at this point it was just too hard to try and write it, to make any sense of my experiences. There was not much time at all for me to have to myself. Looking after Jasper became a full-time job as he became more unwell, and my exhaustion, my depression and my fears deepened.

Diary, 28th November 2014

No idea what has been written before now, I'm aware there is a big space – six months or so... I have no idea how to articulate the last three months; harrowing. He is fading and grieving, losing the fight and the will. Sometimes that brings humour but mostly a relentless horror, a fear that I can't begin to write about. I had a proper full-blown panic attack last week, alone at the supermarket; it was awful. I am now at a friend's house having an overnight break. We have been funeral planning, bittersweet moments of pure love and trying so hard, so very hard to be brave. Trying to hold him in the light and carry him forward to where he needs to go. No way back from here, only forward, only through it. I'm reading The Tibetan Book of Living and Dying; it's inspirational and leaves me questioning everything. Everything is in flux and there is no future, that is my belief. No future in that it is unknown, not that I believe it will not happen. We are craving now for the end. The end of this suffering; my gorgeous, lovely gentleman, my love, my beautiful man, you are so thin. My heart, his heart, our hearts are broken; there are no words to describe, to qualify, this experience.

Facebook post, 19th November 2014

The bastard cancer has been kicking our arses lately and Jasper is taking some time out at the Marie Curie Hospice in Edinburgh, to get some symptom control sorted. He isn't up for visitors yet, but is happy to be there, and is being extremely well looked after. Amazing team on hand and a lovely single room. Sending out love and feeling it too. He will be in for a few more days, anyway: ground floor, Room 6, if you're a card-sending type.

Facebook post, 20th November 2014

I have cancelled my Canary Islands holiday next week till things settle down again. The holiday company, Alpharooms, have been great: full refund on my hotel. Ryanair – what are the chances? xx

Facebook post, 29th November 2014

What an incredibly tough couple of weeks we have just been through. Jasper is home from hospice and doing OK. Today I am giving thanks to the folks who came part of the way with us and the utterly amazing staff at Marie Curie. Today I am concentrating on positive love and sending it out, particularly to anyone who has no willingness to try to understand the pain others may be feeling. Happy Saturday, folks; have a love-filled weekend. x

Facebook post, 1st December 2014

Having a wee solo budget break at the Scotsman Hotel; booked the cheapest room on a special deal... So, imagine my surprise to arrive and find a kind and, so far, anonymous person had credited my account with a spa treatment... and imagine my sheer delight to find myself upgraded for free to the BARON SUITE! I have two bathrooms, two TVs, a dining table, another dining table, and the most amazing views across Edinburgh. Let the sleeping and eating begin. Thanks universe. xx

Diary, 2nd December 2014
(another couple of nights' break in a local hotel)

Who could have known it would be so lonely, but so hard to convey? I want to see people, but my world has shrunk so much. I have nothing to talk about except the situation I am in… and I don't want to talk about it because there really is so little to say. It's a horrific nightmare. But this dichotomy; I can't be alone, I can't be with people is paralysing and this extreme I'm in – no brain, sorrow, fear, anger – makes it all pretty hard to reach out and also to be around; I know this to be true. It's natural to want to be alone; it's how I spend that time, though… what shall I do, how will I get through? It has to be a new life, somewhere far from here and this pain. How can I remain here after he has gone? I yearn for it. Watching my love fade and disappear before me has changed me beyond all recognition. I don't know some of my old pals any more; they don't feel part of this for me now. Maybe that's natural, or maybe some of them just can't be what I need.

Facebook post, 5th December 2014

I'm really not on here much these days, except to be flippant about holiday breaks. Thanks for asking after us. I'm full of a cold this week, and, as ever, I am running to stand still, just trying to keep all the plates spinning; juices, shopping, housework, medications, but we have our gorgeous lady Sue about to arrive to help us plan Christmas. (Baubles, anyone? Yes, we know, the secret's out, and we love you all deeply for it, you crazy, beautiful people – it's going to have to be a two-tree Christmas; you can admire your handiwork on the 28th, Miss Daisy.) We are muddling along, it's up and down, and we are doing what we can, when we can... today's been a good day. LOVE. LOVE. LOVE. xx

Diary, 13th December 2014

He is sleeping more and more and looking a bit more at peace at times. What a struggle he is having, my lovely love; his pain is still increasing, and he is still losing weight. I'm sleeping in the front room as I have had an awful cold, but I am visiting our bed at bedtimes to hold him, and sometimes in the night I wake and rush through, because I just need to be right beside him; the fear I will find him passed away is always with me. I am trying to reside in that place 'above' or 'beside' the knowing he won't be here, quite soon. He just won't be here. It's too hard. I can't engage with it; it will break me. I must remain strong, for us both.

This morning I woke up thinking about names and what they mean. If I keep my name, my married name, will I remain a person who will always be bereaved? Always a widow? There must be a new start at some point; maybe a new name would be ideal. The old me is dying alongside my husband. I don't know who I am any more. I have been profoundly changed by this loss. Our loss. I don't know how I can ever fall in love again – I feel I could not betray him that way, and I could not risk this pain. I want to find joy in myself, not another person, first and foremost, and that must be my mission. To heal my body and my mind.

Diary, 17th December 2014

Golden days, light, filled with love these past two days; he is in good spirits and almost like his old self. We are cuddling and smooching and caring and holding and laughing and dancing and naming each joy as it comes. Golden. I am so happy he is finding more peacefulness, happy that he can look outward and feel joy, feel love. What a dark time it's been since September. He is frailer day by day but for now anyway his soul is light and I'm so grateful to see the man I love so dearly. It's wonderful to find him again, shining out in amongst all that pain, that untold pain.

Facebook post, 20th December 2014

Wishing all the lovely family and pals a very gorgeous sherry mishmash. It's golden and warm and cosy and 'koselig' here. The baubles are still arriving through the post, the tree is mighty! I am not on Facebook much at all at the minute but doing OK, and much better this week, with a bit of hands-on help from our friends. Looking forward to a very snug and homey festive season. Today we made it to the beach for the first time in months... and here's that tree and its growing story. xx

Diary, 26th December 2014

Boxing Day – another midnight admission by ambulance due to deep trauma and pain in his legs; the spinal cancer has gotten a hold now. Sue, Roy and Lindsay are with us for Christmas. Jasper went in on crutches 'cause the ambulance men brought the wrong type of ambulance with no stretcher – who could have known that when you ring an ambulance, an emergency ambulance, you need to have the presence of mind to request a 'two-man stretcher ambulance'? I was so angry; they were all set to bump him down three flights of stairs in a wheelchair. I flipped and cried out to them, "Spinal tumours, cord compression, paralysis!" I am always fighting, fighting, fighting for him, the worst time so far, and I am there, curled up on a makeshift bed in the corner of his tiny room, overnight, there 90% of the time.

Facebook post, 30th December 2014

Just for your info, folks, Jasper is currently having a hospice stay to get some symptom control sorted. He is up for visitors. Marie Curie Hospice, Frogston Road, Liberton, Room 5, first floor. He has some hospital stuff coming up from Tuesday so message us before setting out on the Number 11 bus in case he's not here!

Marino Branch
Brainse Marino
Tel: 8336297

Facebook post, 31st December 2014

A bittersweet year of extreme difficulty and extreme love.
A year of strengthening true friendships and kindnesses
from unexpected places, and profound changes within. Be
well, be kind. xx

Marie Curie was our hospice and the staff there got to know us well. They always did the best they could for us, and I will be forever grateful for their care, although at times it seemed frustratingly slow while they spent days adjusting meds and waiting to see if they had it right before sending him home. They got to know that if Jasper scored three out of ten on a pain chart – they would always ask, "What is your level of pain out of ten, with ten being the worst?" and he would always say three – and then they would glance at my face and back to him, before asking again, this time he might concede a four or five. And we would all know he really meant a seven.

Some staff became favourites whom Jasper trusted, and if they could, these nurses, Martin in particular, would spend time with him during panic attacks, holding his hand, trying to talk him down, allowing me an hour to drive home, shower, change my clothes and try to eat something, although there was rarely anything appetising; I was at the hospice so much the fridge was empty and the cupboards bare. I could order and pay for meals at the hospice, but they had to be ordered twenty-four hours previously and most of the time, I couldn't think that far ahead. All concern for my health and well-being was gone. All I could think of was Jasper and our 'journey', and when would it end? I longed for the end. I was utterly terrified of it, afraid of the pain he might suffer, but I longed for the peace of not being needed twenty-four hours a day, week in, week out, month after month, with no end in sight. It was a living hell.

Most hospice rooms were large and airy, some with balconies or access to outside. We experienced quite a few of them. It is a strange, hushed world, the world of the dying. It became our second home, so much so I could sometimes bypass the on-call GP – by whom you had to be referred to be admitted – and phone the ward direct. If they had a bed, I could take Jasper in.

During the nightmare that became Christmas 2014, we spent three weeks in the hospice, in several different rooms. Jasper was in agony, as the cancer had found its way around the Tarceva and spread to his pelvis and spine. I cannot begin to imagine how he suffered during this time, although I was ever present and some nights in such despair and terror at his pain levels, I begged the doctors to make him pain free. That was what we had been promised by our Marie Curie nurse; he didn't need to be in pain. However, to give him ketorolac, an injectable anti-inflammatory, only allowed once a day due to bleed-out risk, he had to come off the Tarceva. It was the beginning of the end. His lung cancer became active again.

I stayed at the hospice with him, on camp beds and sofas, or sleeping in armchairs, with a blanket over me, ready to call for help when the next wave hit. A horrific time, which broke us further and has scarred me mentally; I cannot shake these images from my mind. They repeat and repeat and give me no peace; they find me in twisted dreams and night terrors. All the 'whys' and 'ifs' and 'how I could have done better'. I know I was a nightmare – a ball of exhaustion, fear and stress, and stretched so tight I would snap at the slightest thing. There were times he hated me – a manifestation of the total dependency he now had on me. He couldn't manage without me, and he hated that and the strain it put on me; he could see me breaking, as I saw it in him, and it tested us sorely.

During this time, it was decided he needed radiotherapy to try to reduce the pressure on his spine from the tumours. I was to take him in the car from the hospice to the Western General on the other side of the city. He was so claustrophobic by now that the car was too small, and he would come out of near-catatonic states to struggle with door handles as he tried to exit the car as we were moving. He was driven by such terror of the small space that he just didn't care about or see the danger he was in. Even dosed up on lorazepam to try and keep him calm, I was pretty sure he wouldn't be able to lay on the radiotherapy bed, completely still for long minutes, and bear the solitude and fear while the beams hit. I had experienced weeks of this the previous summer, and I knew how hard it was. He couldn't be left alone due to panic and I wasn't allowed in with him while the beam was going; the door would be locked.

The clinics were closed for Christmas and it was surreal to arrive at the seemingly empty department – doors locked, ring a bell and a radiologist nurse would appear and let us in. Jasper, catatonic with fear in a hospital wheelchair, me struggling to pull him along – damn those things – was supposed to have three sessions over five days. He managed one – and that night was hell; radiotherapy is not painless and can initially cause 'tumour flare'. He steadfastly refused to go back. We nearly made it the next day – I got him as far as the radiotherapy suite, but to no avail.

He was also supposed to have a brain scan somewhere around this time, but it was out of the question. Our options were becoming extremely limited due to his panic attacks and claustrophobia.

Jasper had several hospice admissions over the winter. Sometimes it was for pain, which was extreme and required radiotherapy. He also required a new drug which could not be used with the Tarceva, due to the danger of internal bleeds. In the end we didn't have to make the awful decision to stop the Tarceva, knowing it would mean the beginning of the end. The cancer made that decision for us, and by now, Jasper was saying he had had enough. These were such dark days and sometimes he would be admitted to hospice for the terrible anxiety which now ravaged his mind. It was the worst of times and although our love held true, it was pushed to the outer limits of coping, the outer edges of our sanity. I wished it to be over. For both of us.

Facebook post, 4th January 2015

My head's been exploding recently. Today I mused on what I have learnt this week:

I NEED music…

Cucumber makes any juice taste really fine, even the really bogging ones…

When you call an ambulance, you have to state, "Two-man stretcher needed" or they turn up with all the wrong stuff, but don't tell you that's what you needed to say…

People moan about such inconsequential things…

It's extremely humbling to realise life still goes on around you, even when you're not taking part.

Facebook's full of inane chat… this is my contribution.

Facebook post, 8th January 2015

Just to let you know, Jasper is back in Marie Curie at Liberton, in from last Friday morning for symptom control. We're not sure how long he will be in and he is very dopey at times, but he is very happy to have visitors in his teeny-tiny room. Please text ahead to make sure he's still there. Number 11 bus goes all the way from Leith Walk through town and stops right outside, both directions. And… if you could send a virtual Mexican wave of love I would be very appreciative indeed.

As things progress and as we move from the general to the particular, our stuff becomes less easy to share here on Facebook. It's been a really hard six months with different crises, and it's been quite impossible to articulate here. Facebook's become a bit daunting really and I am easily overwhelmed. Thanks for the messages, folks. Lots of love. x

Diary, 25th January 2015

What a week of visitors – on and on they come; they come to say goodbye, they leave saying, "See you soon." They come back, to say goodbye again. Another tough day today with Jasper in the deepest doldrums and me unable to do anything but sit and be with him, encourage the pill-taking and just hold him through it. Jem turned up and he immediately brightened; he's now out for a walk with Lenka and it's a small space for me to scribble in. I hate my life, simple and true. I need a place to feel safe, to be able to make sense of it all. I need to write about what is happening to us, but it is more difficult than I can possibly articulate. I am utterly exhausted, overwhelmed and claustrophobic; there is nothing but this awful focus on cancer. Jasper is completely consumed by it, no room for my troubles; he has become utterly selfish, in its purest form. When he does talk to me it is only in reference to himself – emotions, eating, sleeping, grumping, pain, emotions, no emotions, a paralysis of emotions.

This entry distressed me hugely; I sound so selfish. I know it's partly that the diary entries are the hard end of everything, and they don't tell the whole story. But I'm deeply upset that I couldn't give more than I did, although I know I gave everything. At times he didn't want anything from me. Just seeing my face made his broken heart tear further. I couldn't possibly hide my devastation. We knew each other too well for such disguises.

My next diary entry is a bit odd. It's eight things about cancer – obviously, I am raging inside my confines:

Diary 1st February 2015

1. *Cancer doesn't care, but it's dark and cruel.*
2. *It's a clever wee thing and it will find a way around most strategies.*
3. *It's so clever it creates its own blood supply – creepy, really creepy.*
4. *Cancer has many causes. My belief? A mix of circumstance and environmental poisoning; both of us were living in the 'red zone' on the map of fallout for Chernobyl in 1984; me in Scottish Borders, Jasper in Cumbria. Plastic also has its part to play.*

5. *If it's about statistics – well, 100% of our household is affected. Go figure; we are living in an epidemic.*
6. *Marie Curie and Maggie's Centres – what amazing charities. Go fundraise.*
7. *Cancer isolates people. Don't be scared, say hello!*
8. *Doctors give prognoses that people then live by. Live in the present, not in the waiting room.*

Diary, 2nd February 2015

Walking fine lines between what I require for my basic needs – sleeping, eating, juices, exercise, time with friends – and wider needs: a job, fun, adventure, travel, building dreams. They all wait for the one thing I don't ever want to happen; they can only truly begin after that awful thing happens. What a fine line I walk; the balance is impossible; I fall over a lot. We are both waiting for that final moment, both afraid, but for different reasons. He is afraid of death, and I am afraid of how that will be for me and the times to come without him. I am a coper, these past three years have shown me that, but I can't start coping with living without him when he is still here and needs me, so much more than he has ever done. It diminishes us both and is taking a terrible toll on us. There are a lot of days I wish myself dead. These are bad days for sure. There are days when I feel an occasional tiny thrill for a future that can have room for me, and I feel so guilty too – time to write, time to just be, time to create, but the guilt is overwhelming. The thing about cancer is that no one can tell you how it will change you as a person. Today my daughter and I are supposed to be flying off to Tenerife for her twenty-fifth birthday – I am glad we are not going, it's way too stressful. So instead I'm taking her to a posh hotel in Glasgow for two whole glorious nights of no stress, no pain, no injections, and no cancer.

The above is my last diary entry for many months, and Facebook posts alone give me any idea of my situation in the times that followed. While the diary tells the darkest sides, the Facebook posts are a positive spin on the hardest of times. Memory walks a path somewhere in between.

Facebook post, 2nd March 2015

This is a wee shout-out to the pals, steadfast and true, who regularly check in to check up. I'm not mentioning names; you know who you are. Special thanks to the Monday guy, who's pretty much given us every Monday night since early December so I can go to Maggie's Centre, to the other Monday guys who have also stepped in, to my Acorn, for all the compassion and mighty virtual and real hugs, and to those folks with the big house on the hill, who put up our out-of-towners… see, it's hard to stop now. SO much gratefulness and appreciation. THANK YOU. xx

Facebook post, 4th March 2015

Turns out The Beatles were wrong. Love isn't all you need. Needed also are rest and recuperation, space and solitude. I'm having a break next week. I'm seeking cosy, quiet, empty houses, not too far from Edinburgh. I have no chat and no energy to pretend I have chat, and I have no money for a hotel... Just wondering if anyone can help with some free accommodation, with no chat. Thanks. xx

Facebook post, 17th March 2015

ARG!!! OK, big ask coming up... our house is unliveable till Monday 23rd/Tuesday 24th March. We must be in Edinburgh – Southside preferred – to access our community support team. We are not able to camp on floors as Jasper is too poorly with pain. We need a house or flat for a few days, somewhere quiet. Currently in Peebles but have been advised by our Marie Curie nurse we need to be in Edinburgh. ARG!!! Can you help please? PM me if you can help. xx

Facebook post, 21st March 2015

What a crazy, challenging few days, in what is an already very challenging time! Thanks to the lovely folks who have gifted us this safe and lovely place to be. We are safe and sound in lovely sunny Leith, a gorgeous wee flat on the shore. Acorn is cooking up a storm in the kitchen, our fave biking courier Dolphin Boy saving the day with Jasper's much-needed meds. And breathe! Oh, and we've only gone and hit the £2,000 mark for the money we are raising for Maggie's Centres! xx

Facebook post, 27th March 2015

Last week we had to move out of our flat due to our bathroom flooding the downstairs neighbours. Today I have come home to find a large water stain spreading across our kitchen ceiling. The boys upstairs have just had a plumber in doing some work... I am now going to go drink all the gin and then all the wine. That's all.

Although there were many times spent in hospice over that awful last winter, we also had long spells of time at home, and during these times we were blessed to be visited by friends and family. Looking back at the wall calendar I am amazed to see just how busy our flat was. There were the folks from far away; Sarah, Mike and Jude, Martin and Kit, Lucy and Ben, to mention a few, who came to say goodbye, sometimes more than once. There were the folks from nearby; Andy, Suzy, Ali and Lindsey, Donald and Mary, Lenka, Jenny, Rick, Phil, Heather and Vini, and the other friends and our families, who came to support us so I could simply nip to the shops or collect medication. They also came so I could take a couple of days'

break. It was so incredibly hard to let go of that responsibility. I had become habituated to constant worry and it never really left me; I was only ever a phone call and short drive away. Hotel receptionists were told to page me any time, day or night, if I received a call from home. If staying with friends, they were instructed to wake me any time. I rang home several times a day. I remember Jasper's friends coming from afar, one of whom was Daz, a nurse practitioner, and the other his best pal Dave, also an avid sports fan. Jasper and I were both so happy. I could take a break, knowing all aspects were covered. He could enjoy company, watch and chat about sport, and, importantly, he also knew his basic medical care, like injections, or keeping an eye on infections, was covered.

I've no idea how we would have coped without this care and I will be forever grateful to have been so held in the light through such a lonely time. Make no mistake, just because you can't seem to connect with people, because your situation is too far away from their own field of experience, it doesn't mean you don't need to have folks near. Yes, it accentuates the strangeness, but it also means you have some measure of just how far out there you really are. And, importantly, you also have people to bear witness, to see the depths of the struggle and the pain.

During the last twelve weeks of Jasper's life, I was in charge of all his injections, which towards the end were upwards of eighteen per day. However, because they were controlled drugs, we could only have twenty-four hours supply at a time. It became part of the daily routine, and worry, to call the surgery, talk to the GP, order prescriptions, make sure it got to the chemist, make sure they had the drugs in stock, all before the chemist closed. I injected into a butterfly line he had put in on his upper arm at the hospice; but sometimes the butterfly failed or the injection spilled. I had to keep careful note of everything I gave him on a chart. We were terrified of overdose. The day we arrived home back into our flat after the flooding, we were called immediately back into hospice. It was now the end of March. Even with all the medication we couldn't control the pain, and the increasing number of injections was too much for him to have unsupervised. If he died at home, with the amount I was injecting, there would have to be an inquiry, I would be investigated.

He died a week later in the hospice, he was forty four years old. He died in my arms, with his parents at his bedside, as I sang to him through my tears, trying to reassure him, telling him he was loved, he had lived an amazing life filled with laughter and love; telling him we would find each other again. Reminding him he had spread joy around the world, and it was OK for him to go. I would be fine. My daughter and I washed his body and laid him out. I stayed a while, holding his hands, kissing his forehead, wailing in my grief, talking to him, trying to impress his image on my memory, quite unable to leave him. Leaving him there to be collected by the undertaker was the hardest walk I have ever taken. Now I feel dreadful that I left him alone; I realise I could have waited until the undertaker came, and I wish I had. I had no idea; I was so broken.

It was in April 2015 when he left us, on Good Friday. He was in pain until the last, but so far under with the drugs he was no longer able to talk or even squeeze my hand. The images of his last few days and hours were lodged deep in my brain and overlaid everything for many months. They still do at times. Along with those images came the guilt I felt at not being a better wife, at not fixing him, at wanting it to be over for him, at him dying and me living on without him. I still live with this guilt every day. Sometimes it is like a hammer that batters my consciousness in the night, in the day, in the supermarket, in company. No one can see it, but it's there and it will always be there. Such is the widow's lot. The survivor, the one left behind. In the end, although he got two years and four months of living after his diagnosis, the last six months of that time was truly a living hell. No one can prepare you for this scenario, this waiting to die, and in many ways it broke us.

After April 2015

Freefall, spinning, no coherent thought processes, no strength in my legs or body, shaking, sleepless. So terribly shocked. I have no appetite; I swing between no feeling and too much feeling. The world is at a standstill or the world is spinning. Lost. So afraid. So disconnected. So alone. Where are you?

I have horrible panic attacks, my grief is too big, and it doesn't fit into my body. I shake and cry and can't breathe, my legs and hands go numb. I fear I will lose my mind; I have never had this level of attacks before. I am not strong anymore. I am broken. I have no idea when they will hit and so I live in fear of the fear of them. I wander through our flat, sleepless, unable to eat, wearing your big jumper. I am seeing you in every room, laughing, joking, crying, fading, holding on.

Your funeral was a huge affair; it sprouted legs and ran away with you. Our community pulled out all the stops; we rocked the church, over 350 people attended. I talked for many minutes about you and our love and life together. I don't know what gave me the strength, apart from my will to do the best for you. The congregation gave me a standing ovation. You would have been so proud of us, and me, my love.

It was different than we had planned, but it was immense. The street band, New Orleans style, was thirty strong (we had asked for seven musicians). They played you down the street, from the home that we had shared for all those years, to the church around the corner. I remember Heather taking my hand and leading me to our bay window and telling me to look down at your hearse waiting on the street for us; holding me and gently saying I should try to absorb the shock of seeing it and all it meant, and to take a moment to gather my courage. The band played 'I'll Fly Away' and they sang, and the cortège who also walked with you sang, and it lifted me up and it carried me along as I walked behind your hearse. Bystanders clapped and the people in cars, traffic jammed until we passed, cried and clapped too. Acorn and Kit stood by my side all day. Suzy and Heather also carried me when my legs gave way.

I'm so glad we did most of the planning together. We visited the funeral home at the end of our street together. We talked to the funeral director together. I heard recently that you were also given a standing ovation as your coffin left the church. It made me so proud of you to hear this. I did not see or hear it at the time; by then I was in a completely panicked mess, hiding from the congregation, unable to deal with anyone talking to me, hiding in my parents' car, waiting to drive to the crematorium, oh, horror on horror. I am crushed beyond measure. It's so lonely here without you. Where are you?

The 1st May and I am still reeling from exhaustion, stress and loss. I am utterly bewildered; my legs don't work. I can't function. The days drift by in a cloud of grief. I had no idea the body shock would be so huge again. You and I, we anticipated your passing, almost daily, for months, yet it hits like it was never real. Nothing can prepare someone for the absence a death leaves behind. We may know it intellectually beforehand but it makes no sense. None. How can a person who was living and breathing no longer be here? Where are you?

I receive an email from our landlords on 1st May, two weeks after your funeral. Eviction. The house will be put on the market in eight weeks. I am shocked to my already broken core. On the same day, I also receive a handwritten letter from a friend on the Hebridean island where we spent so many years. Would I like to house-sit for a month in July? It seems I have no choice. I must pack up our home, downsize it to make it fit into my parents' garage, and move to the island. I will stay a month in Berni's house, then move into our tiny six-by-eight-foot caravan. I am homeless.

I don't know how I get through the awful eight weeks that follow as I sift and sort through our life. At a time when I think I can finally collapse, spend days in bed, drinking too much and grieving loudly, this is not to be. I am once more deferring my needs. I have too much to do. Friends come and take away furniture and plants. Ali and Lindsey remove the massive daily pile of junk, to the charity shops and the dump, from the hall where I pile it up. Mary and Donald come and take away your ashes, for safekeeping. I cannot bear to look at them. They represent a horror I can never have anticipated. Mary also packs up your clothes and puts them safe. Apart from your jumper, which I am wearing constantly, and sleep curled around at night. I can't look at your clothing, it hurts too much.

Somewhere in this time I realise I must deal with your grow rooms. They are empty of plants but need to be cleaned and dismantled. The dried bud is lined up and awaiting a cook. How can I find the strength to do this alone? I call in yet another favour and I take it all, plus the cooking equipment, out to the countryside. I and a friend cook up your many months of careful growing. I have not the wherewithal to order more isopropyl, so we use the tiny amount I have brought with me. It's not enough.

The bud is hardly covered; still we persevere, mashing it up hard, rinsing and rinsing again. She carefully puts the stuff we would normally throw away to one side and says she will do another cook once she has ordered more iso. We do well, but only manage to get around thirty grams of oil.

I take it home for the final stage, that slow burning off of the last remnants of the iso. It's a stage that can take twenty-four hours, and an infrared thermometer is a good tool to acquire as it saves guesswork and many hours. The flat is stinking with it and I'm very afraid someone will notice. We always managed to OD at this point, in our previous cooks, and once again I forget the potency. As I'm drawing it up into the syringes the waste seems crazy, and absent-mindedly I lick the ends of the syringes. Much too late I realise I have had at least twenty-five times the recommended starting dose. I haven't had any oil for months and I have no tolerance at all. A friend is round for dinner and I try to serve her chicken, which is raw apart from the outer edges, which fortunately she notices, and I put it back in the frying pan. I am desperate to get her to leave before I start tripping. I have no idea what will happen, and I am very frightened. As she leaves, I find I cannot even stand up. I'm desperately pretending I'm OK, that I am just tired. She has no idea of what I have done to myself. I'm glad; there's no way she would have left if she had known. I lie on the couch. I try very hard to focus my mind away from grief. I cannot bear to go to the dark place in the state I am about to be in. I find my body beginning to tense; my system is fully overloaded. My central nervous system is twitching and shaking, and I keep shouting out and making strange groaning noises. I am deeply afraid. Do I need to be hospitalised? What on earth would I say? Even if I could talk, how could I begin to explain what I've done and what's happening to me? I try to stand up again and cannot. I crawl to the bathroom and realise I must try to get to bed and sleep if I can. All the while I am keeping my grief at bay, holding it tight. It cannot be allowed to be a part of this trip. I crawl to my bed and somehow climb up and into it. I lay there and think to myself, *I will wait five minutes and if I don't fall asleep I will take two sleeping pills and try to just get through the night in one piece.* Somewhere deep inside I know you would be alternately laughing at me and scolding me for being so daft.

I wake the next morning, thankful I am alive. I try to stand and find I still can't walk. I spend the rest of that day and some of the next completely stoned, flaked out and sleeping deeply. In the days that follow I develop a very sore and itchy rash all over my body. My hands are particularly bad, and I realise I am toxic. My liver is working very hard to rid my body of the oil. I am very shaken by this experience. The next time I see my friend who helped me cook, she hands me another thirty grams from the third rinse with the already washed bud. We did it; we made a full treatment. She also tells me she's taken some and has journeyed to meet her ancestors. She believes it to be very powerful and pure medicine, likening it to peyote or ayahuasca.

I move to the island on 2nd July, in a complete daze, stunned, heartsore, broken and weary to my bone, and, unbeknownst to me, I am already nursing a broken rib, with more on the way. The island folks meet me, and I am enveloped into a small community who know about grief. Everyone I see makes sure to speak directly to me. I have developed a phobia about seeing people for the first time and I am hugely relieved to be somewhere where folks seem to understand it's best to just greet the bereaved, say hello and then that part is done. I am also relieved there is a finite amount of people here, only around one hundred, compared to the city. The randomness of suddenly bumping into someone who I have not seen since you died is no longer an issue. I begin to breathe again. My panic lessens and an overwhelming exhaustion begins to hit. I sleep. I sleep a lot.

My first diary entry is very short; I am drunk.

Diary, 10th August 2015

Our caravan on Eigg, rain, six weeks nearly since I arrived here and I am trying to write for the first time since February. This is made very difficult due to whisky and grief. WTF can I even say about grief? Empty. Sad.

Diary, 12th (?) August 2015

Eigg. Like the sheer cliffs that I gaze at, across the flat Minch, my grief seems unscalable – waves crash, sometimes for days, but they don't impact, they don't break through the holding pattern I have developed. I fear my coping strategy may be the end of me.

Diary 14th August 2015

My world is lived through analogy and space. There are too many spaces that are my husband's shape. Some days you are here, so close, my love, it's almost unbearable, it is unbearable, but somehow I bear it. Do I? Well, I get through and it begins again. I can feel the next storm rising – its signals are endless ruminating on stuff, increased anxiety, proneness to uncontrollable weeping, lack of care for myself and lack of food. The storm will break, somehow, and I will begin again at numbness – the default, the welcome, awful default.

A life lived through analogies 'cause there are no actual words of mine to describe the missing of my heart, my soulmate – no way to articulate how memory slams me; assailed some days, minute to minute, with full-size, Technicolor you, and I feel so blessed to have them and I try to ride them and 'see you'. I SEE YOU! But then the awfulness of loss slams in again and I am lost again, and so it goes on. My soul roars for you and I hope you cannot hear me – I fear it will only cause you pain. I believe you are everywhere and nowhere. You are in everything, but you are not here. Where are you? This is what my soul roars. Where are you, my love?

I have been here six weeks now and I feel I am no further forward. Life is as simple as I want it to be. The caravan is a blessing and I'm so lucky to have that place to be. Damian, bless him, you would be so proud of His Palship, my husband; he has strimmed the head-high jungle and tangle of briars and grasses that were right up to our caravan door, made me a stile to climb onto the croft with, and is today building a composting toilet with Dougie. How amazing.

Wes has been so generous to let me have this time here. I wrote him a card today and put some of your herbs in it, then I ran away. I am so shy of him and Maggie.

And here I am, 'sat sitted' in full sun, bra and pants, best day of the summer. I hope the weather holds and I will see the gorgeous sunset and maybe the last of the Perseid meteor shower. And so I count my blessings, and there you are in the sky, beaming warmth and comfort onto my body and soul. Will I always live a life in the extremes? I want simple things now you're not here to adventure with me. I think I want to remain here.

Several times over the course of that dark and wet summer I had occasion to believe very much in the power of the spirit that becomes energy. I repeatedly cried out for my husband. From the bottom of my soul I cried, *Where are you?* and often the sun would choose that moment to burst through and catch me in its rays.

I remember sitting outside the caravan, searching in my mind for him. Suddenly ahead of me a tree branch began to shake and shake and shake. I watched and wondered. I moved closer and strained to see the creature that surely was responsible for this happening. I couldn't find it. In the end I went back to my chair and accepted my belief – he was there with me, in a form of pure energy, and this was his way of saying hello.

Another time, a few days later, I'm in the same position outside the van. It's a rare day of sunshine, one of only five we have over a very wet eight weeks. I am sitting very still, lost in my thoughts, and wondering and musing on loss and the sublime. Unexpectedly, right in front of my face there appears a huge orange-and-black dragonfly – its wings are so big they span my face and it's literally two inches from the end of my nose and making an intense whirring sound. I laugh out loud at the cheekiness of it and the joy to have nature so close. It flies away, and the next thing I find, it has landed on my upper arm; it's several inches long and is looking at me. My every instinct is to swat it; I'm a bit frightened it may bite me. It's huge. It sits, we stare at each other for a minute, and then it takes off. I laugh again and take a breath. Then it's back. It's in my face, whirring away. This process repeats six times; in my face, on my arm. I feel light-headed and bit crazy, but I believe Jasper is here with me. Somehow. This experience will stay with me forever. I have never seen a dragonfly this size, nor heard of one behaving like this. Call me crazy. I'm happy with that. I later find out that dragonflies are considered to be the doorway between worlds.

Diary, 18th (?) August 2015

Eigg – such shifts and changes, feeling very alone now, would like to be included more in the community here. I am welcomed and accepted if I arrive places, but getting out the door alone is hard.

I wrote the above, and as I wrote feeling very alone the blue tea-light holder fell off the shelf...

It's good to be writing again; something has shifted there. I feel stuck a lot of the time, day to day, with the decisions I need to make 'cause there is no one to talk them over with. I'm too fragile and I want to be calm and find my place, locate myself in my location. Maybe this is why I am here: to slow down, to be simple, to re-energise and grow, not to drink whisky and smoke and fall over. I need to sit right here in nature and let myself be soothed by the sublime. I should be reading the romantics – Coleridge, your time has come.

I am planning on leaving here two weeks on Tuesday. Today I woke wanting to leave. It's the first time really, and I had to remind myself I have no home to go to. Literally. The city doesn't appeal. I thought about heading south to Towersey Festival; Jasper's public tribute is the day after my birthday and I would love to be there with all the old crowd, but I couldn't stand the rubbernecking from the public so... maybe next year, and maybe there will be work there for me too. Maybe I will get back to performing. I am enjoying the wee bits of singing I do here at events. There are so many reasons to stay here and only one reason to go: that is, I miss talking with my friends and I am not doing well at keeping in touch. There is no phone signal at the caravan. It is hard to remember to charge up my phone when I'm living without electricity, and maybe I should put my answerphone on again.

Diary, no date; sometime in August 2015

Still in the caravan – I'm beginning to feel a rhythm to my days: get up early, potter and tidy the tiny space; clean out the stove, chop wood, collect water, wash the dishes, eat breakfast if I'm in good form, and then off to work. Drive across the hill to Kildonan, and always I am taken aback by the beauty of the vista, no matter the weather – providing I can see a few feet in front of me. Get to work, gossip with Marie, clean the B&B, change beds, scrub bathrooms. Tea and cake with Marie, more chat.

Afternoons are variable depending on whether I need to go to the shop or not. I enjoy the afternoon sun here on the croft, and when it gets too shady I head down to my favourite spot on the beach. No one can see me from here, and I gaze at the water, looking for signs – always looking for signs – and looking for dolphins and whales. The tide is high at about 7pm and it's the best time for the beach.

Today I found myself explaining to Berni, as she cooked us lunch, about the decision to stop the Tarceva so we could use the drug that it interacts badly with, and how it meant the loss of hope, really. It struck me how much I have forgotten about the horrors that I have seen and been fully, fully involved in – some horrible decisions, all made through the veil of psychological and physical exhaustion. Do I feel guilty? Always. Did I do my best? Nearly always. Meh.

I have also realised this will always be in me – this place I share with you. It requires solitude.

I also need to talk to others, though, to work it out, this horror, let it come to the fore. My journey home is booked. I will now make a Maggie's appointment and an appointment with Susana, book lots of dinners with pals, and I need to try to be true to what I really need.

Friday? I have lost the date now… part of my free fall. Another night of heavy rain all night long. This is the worst summer (official) for one hundred years. My, oh my, and I live in a space which is six-by-eight feet. Maybe we will all float away, or sink into the Atlantic with all the rain, rain, rain.

I feel I have wasted some of my time here. Lost days due to drinking or simply having no energy; maybe the above is crap and all has been as it should be. 'Home' in only ten days. The city and people and a new space to try to create a home in. A home, alone. That will keep me busy. I don't know if I can cope with the stress of it all, though. I'm going to soak up the sublime over this last bit of time. Sit on the beach, go walking. The new composting toilet is fantastic; well done, Damian and Dougie, what stars. Must get Damian some nice whisky, and some cash too for materials.

Diary, 30th August 2015

On the mezzanine at Damian's. It's my forty eight birthday. I have been dreading this day, just as I dreaded yours back in July, my love. I am sat up in bed, still in my jim-jams, some lovely cards from folks and a brilliant set of presents from my daughter, bless her! So good to have something to open. She is a total honey. Feeling OK, not too wobbly or emotional, but hung-over – whisky in the pub till very late last night. Heading to the shower and then off to meet Sarah, and then to Berni's for some food. Feeling happy.

The island has been very tough; it was always going to be so. But it has also been very isolating to be so far from my close friends and my family. I am utterly toxic from all the whisky and I have taken up smoking again after twelve years of not smoking. It's crazy. I have no care for myself. I can hardly breathe and I suspect I have several broken ribs, or possibly my cancer has run rife through me and my time is near. I can't think straight; it's as though a fog descended over my brain in April and won't lift. I can't remember the last time I could think straight, or think about my needs.

I am dreading returning to our city, the place where we spent so many happy years. I'm moving into Suzy's empty house for a bit. It's a cosy wee two-bedroomed place in the north of the city, far from where we lived. I feel panicked to be leaving the island. It has become home, and although I have spent the summer being quite unable to be in company, unless drunk, it has felt safe and I have found some sort of peace here within the nature and the sublime. I have found you too; in the sun, in the waves, in the big skies and in the dragonflies. I leave the island much as I arrived, utterly broken and distressed. I cry all the way home. I drive on alone through the long commute, down through Glencoe, nursing my sore side and feeling a rising tide of panic.

Back to the City

I arrive back in the city and I am completely lost. I had hoped for a huge welcome, people to meet me, carry me through the first few days of disconnection. But I am alone. Everyone seems busy and as though they have forgotten what we all went through before I left. I am completely unravelled and don't think I have ever felt so alone. I must find the strength to pick up my life and try to begin. But everywhere is a challenge: you are in every petrol station, in every supermarket. I wander hollow-eyed through the city, seeing you at every turn. I have been quite unable to take any oil for months now. It strips away the tiny veneer of coping and I am rocked to my soul by the grief that is waiting to come out at every opportunity. I know I should be taking what we previously called a 'maintenance' dose, a tiny smear every day. But it's utterly impossible; it makes me feel too much. I put it away for another day.

We had made enough for two treatments, and I kind of thought that if I kept taking a tiny dose every day it would protect me, keep my breast cancer at bay. There was no science to this thinking, but I needed to feel I was doing something to protect myself, because I had not taken the oncology drugs or the chemo that were recommended to me.

Diary, 4th September 2015

I slept here last night in a wee nest on the floor and woke up today to sunshine through the windows. The flat is great, very quiet and lots of trees everywhere outside. I am lonely, though; it's Friday now and I've not really heard from people. Guess I need to get out there but it's so hard when I'm so wrecked, emotionally, physically. I managed to get some shopping in today and finally I am able to eat properly; that's been a really tough part of living in the caravan, a very hard part of having to fend for myself and not having the energy to do so... So, food, sleep, write, walk. I live right on the cycle path; it's beautiful, tree-lined, green, and the swimming pool is just five minutes away. God, I couldn't possibly swim, though. My chest wall is truly sore. I am really, really frightened.

Diary, 11th September 2015

Our wedding anniversary – oh, my heart, oh, my sweet love, where are you? The girls came round last night to welcome me to my new home, they are kind and generous with me and my lack of function and my unhappiness, but it just ended up a rammy of whisky-drinking and talking nonsense. I wanted to talk about you, our wedding day, to relive the memories, but it didn't happen and so it became even more lonely than if I'd been here alone. So much lonelier than it needs to be. I'm out of step with this world, I'm bored and restless, I want more than this. I want you. I want a life. I want to be with people who will let me feel and make room for my heart and its breaking. Maybe I hide it too well. I miss you so much. I am now waiting for the person who can come along and sit with me, and when I feel safe, I can ask them, "Have you ever been so lonely you have held your own hand?" This phrase keeps coming back to me. I find myself talking to people and wondering if I could ask such a question. Kit, maybe?

Facebook post, 11th September 2015

My husband, my dear, sweet love. Today is our day. Always and forever. I have no words to express how much I miss you. How deep, how wide. My heart is broken from the missing of you. Such sorrow now on what was such a happy, happy day. Rest easy, my love. Thank you for all the happy days we had together. I will always love you, this day and for all the days to come.

Diary, 14th September 2015

I have gone early to bed. I am enjoying the peaceful, tree-filled view and a striped mauve-and-blue sky. The trees are turning. A lesson learned. I'm done with doing my special big days with people – that was so horrible on Friday; I woke so sad and with no reserves left to deal with the fact it was our wedding anniversary; my first without you. My longing to be with Kit was so powerful. A longing to sit with my friend and look through the wedding albums and talk about our day, eat food and be cared for, and for it to be acknowledged that this is really fucking sore.

In spite of my wretched hung-over state I had a nice day, with meeting Rani for lunch and Jenni scooping me up and feeding me in the morning. Friday morning – our wedding anniversary – was the first time I truly felt like ending my life. I felt I could not bear this pain, this loss. I must try to stay away from that place, and the whisky too. It brings the darkness so much closer. I wander around in my life in a daze of confusion – is this my house? Is this my life? It feels as though I'm just visiting, as though I have fallen down the rabbit hole. I think I have.

I need to mention your name every day, to keep you with us by remembering out loud, reminding folks you existed, that you were once very much part of the tapestry of our lives. You were a thread that ran through communities, out across the wide world. You were a huge presence. I know that folks aren't forgetting you, but I still need to say your name.

Diary, 15th September 2015

I am beginning to feel more at home here in the new flat. The hospital rang yesterday; the lymph node biopsy is tomorrow. Guess it's not unexpected but I would rather it was not yet. Amazing, the capacity to avoid thinking, but it's also very tiring and brings its own silent depression. There was a chart on Facebook this week showing the stages of grief and bereavement – shaped like a U, each stage labelled; shock, denial, anger, bargaining, depression, acceptance, hope, all following the curve of the U. I hadn't realised there were so many stages; however, they had all been joined up, randomly criss-crossing each other with straggly lines that looked like chaos. That made sense to me! Depression is the isolator, though; all the others are more easily... ah, WTF am I saying?

I get the all-clear from the hospital and the results of the recent bone scan: it turns out I have been carrying around three new broken ribs this summer. No wonder I was struggling so hard on the island. I can't believe I worked every day and played my guitar and sang. It was getting very hard to breathe right enough, and I could hardly drive the removal van when we moved my stuff to the new flat. The ribs are broken near my centre, on the right side, and are called 'spontaneous fractures' as they seem to have no cause. They happened during the summer; maybe grief broke them. They are on my radiotherapy side, and are a reason I never wanted that stuff zapped at me. That's now seven broken ribs over two summers. It's amazing, the capacity to just keep going through such physical pain.

Diary, 24th September 2015

This week's been another tough one – Saturday at Al's wedding, mostly OK, but one moment of pure reality when I saw us in another couple dancing with abandon, and I saw us and I broke, right there, I broke in the middle of that dance floor.

I drove to the Lake District the next day and I broke there too, complete teary emotion. Oh my, the missing of you, the really missing, the everyday walking along the street, having a chum, someone to share the chores. Someone to speak with, who understands me like only you did, aw, pal. I miss you. There's another missing, a sudden gut-wrenching twist, and it comes with a memory and it's physical and actually pulls the body, as if it's a time bubble/loop to the happy times. I think this is what happened on Saturday at the wedding. The Lakes were beautiful, stunning, so hot. Dave and Marion scooped me up, such care, such good friends, and I sat outside on Jem's patio, tired and blubbing and unable to look after myself too well, not even to make a sandwich, even though I was very hungry. Marion heard me on the phone to Kit and my plea to make Christmas just disappear, and she invited me to spend it with her and Dave. I'm so pleased. Particularly as I said, "Oh, Marion, what if I just cry all through Christmas?" and she said, "Don't worry, we shall all cry together."

Diary, 3rd October 2015

It will be twenty-six weeks next Friday – six months since you left us – and the missing of you continues to grow. Oh, my love, I miss your tactile being, our hugs, our holds, our wee dances, the way I fit perfectly under your chin, your tender way of holding me so I wouldn't break. I miss our sit-besides, just touching, holding knees, holding toes, holding hands. I miss our cuddling and spooning and nuzzling, heads melding, touching ears and touching necks, and your arms, your lovely, handsome, elegant, beautiful arms. I miss you. Some days are unbearable. My grief is too raw and at the very surface of me, there is no hiding place.

Even though I have been given the all clear at the breast clinic, I feel I should try again to take our cannabis oil, in very small amounts. I think I can use it as a replacement for tamoxifen, which I continue to refuse. This medicine is recommended by my oncologist for me to take for the next ten years, to keep me safe from recurrence, but it's no use, it makes me very unwell. I try it several times, but I am toxic within a few days of taking tamoxifen; I feel fluey and achy and sick to my stomach. The cannabis oil doesn't work for me either; I just end up crying and wandering through the house, restless and bored with myself, but quite unable to reach out and tell my friends and family how much I want my life to end. I consider suicide most days. But it's a futile dream. No one will ever forgive me if I take my own life, and I'm not selfish or desperate enough to really consider it, apart from as a daydream, a choice I think I have, to get me through the very bad days.

Facebook post, 3rd October 2015

Six months. Impossibly, inevitably, today is six months. Today I am sending out loving thoughts and memories of you. I have been thinking a lot recently about how lucky we are to have known you and to have been directly in the beam of your love. Such a gentleman. Always. I have been remembering your cheeky face, your naughty grin, your bad jokes, your balancing ways, your happy patience and your gentleness; been remembering your dancing feet and your juggling arms. Been thinking about your enduring, endearing willingness to do anything for anyone, anywhere, at any time. Such a positive force in so many lives, and always larger than life in ours. I carry you with me every day, my love; we continue to live in the beam.

October 2015

Holiday, solo. Three years and more in the wishing and manifested as a return trip to a gorgeous wee gem of a Venetian port in Crete, where I spent one night at the end of June 2015, during much-needed ten day break with Acorn.

Diary, Wednesday 7th October 2015, Chania, Crete

I have arrived! I am here! First solo travelling for such a long time, and special as I travel alone and also holiday alone. I wonder how I will fare, not speaking to anyone but hoteliers and waiters? How will I fare? How will I fare?

I am excited and flushed with my success. It is an enormous thing to travel alone, and to be alone and to not freak out and get upset and flee from here. To remain calm and to keep my faith in myself and my potential.

My room in Pension Nora has turned into, not the one-room bedsit I'd expected, but a three-storey town house with a balcony on the top floor and a sit-ootery at the front door; it's lush but in a simple Cretan way, well set up and very homely.

The food is poor. Generally. Poor Crete. This is the one, the only, reason I hesitated to return. Ah well, I have a beer in one hand, a cigarette in another (after all, there's only me here, no one to tell me I shouldn't smoke; I feel giddy with the perceived freedom from myself). What will I find out about myself this week; what's it for? A break from being brave... hmmm, not that. A break from the loneliness of Edinburgh – yes, that for sure. And if I'm to be lonely then at least this week it's just down to me.

I'm here!

Glorious, empty, lonely, sun-filled days drift by. I eat, drink, smoke, sleep, wander. I write in my journal all about what's around me. What I can see. Not much on what I feel. I take short breaks from breaking, and it feels sad and so lonely, but right too. I'm supposed to be here; I try to look up, look out, be in the world. This is time for me to just be. To remember how to be.

I keep some contact with home through Facebook posts and begin an unintended blog about what I learn or observe.

Facebook post, 8th October 2015

THINGS I HAVE LEARNT TODAY:

1. *Never, ever, take a woolly jumper to the Mediterranean.*
2. *Always be prepared to haggle. I miss you, husband, and your haggling ways, sometimes to the point of embarrassment for me:*
   > *"It's only 5p, Jasper, why are you asking to make it 3p?"*
   > *"Just for the fun of it, wife!"*
3. *I don't like Cretan food.*
4. *Cretan wine is almost undrinkable.*
5. *Running is totally going to break your feet. Running for a train or a plane is still going to break your feet. Don't run. Don't ever run.* [Every holiday I ever have, it seems, is blighted by some sore feet issue – I write this on 31st January 2016 with sprained ligaments in my right foot, caused by a fall during a minibreak in Glasgow, incorporating a five-hour A&E checking-out session. I hobbled out again in a moon boot and on crutches, – what's it all about? Do my feet just get too itchy?]
6. *Solo travellers make other folk nervous. Hi! Sorry!*
7. *The people staying in the pension opposite can hear me talking to myself.*
8. *Points 3 and 4 cancel each other out. Points 6 and 7 are not related.*
9. *Raki is evil.*

Diary, Friday 9th October 2015

I feel guilty for all the times I didn't hold Jasper tighter, for all the times I was too busy to stop for a hug, a smooch. I wish I could go back and do it all again. I feel guilty that Rani wasn't there right at the end; she missed him leaving us by a few moments, and all for picking up a sandwich for me. I keep seeing your hands and your arms in my mind's eye. Remembering the feel of your paw in mine, and how hard it was to let that hand go. I miss you every single day. I still can't believe you have gone. It's still a shock and it will always be so.

I remember you throwing your head back with laughter – that huge laughter that was contagious and always made me smile, no matter how grumpy I was.

I feel guilty for all the stressing I used to do; so unnecessary. I wish you could see the person your death and our last couple of years have made me become. So much calmer now. It's so clear to me how much time I wasted that could have been better spent. I am sorry, my love. So very sorry.

Today's been a lonely day, for sure. Partly due to meeting an old bloke called David and discussing with him, over breakfast in a cafe, where we shared a table, life as a single person and the loneliness of the state. Or maybe it's just all the alcohol I had yesterday, or the sleeping pill the night before, or maybe because I am in fact lonely. Yip, that's probably it.

Facebook post, 10th October 2015

MORE RANDOM FACEBOOK OBSERVATIONS:

1. *Woman seem more bored with men, than men.*
2. *Woman wear T-shirts with slogans across the front and then give you the evil eye when you're trying to read their message.*
3. *Hot climates are an excuse to dress way below your years.*
4. *There are zillions of long, short dogs in Chania. They are long in body and short in the leg.*
5. *Never feed the cats; there are many and they are feral and they bite.*
6. *Raki is still evil.*
7. *No matter how many questions you ask the waiter, they are so over the season, they don't ask a single one back.*
8. *They (the waiters) are suspicions of me and my note-taking.*

Diary, 10th October 2015

Will there ever come a time when I am not assailed by memories of Jasper? Badminton, laughing, him in a sarong, haggling, swimming – God, the list is endless, and each memory comes unbidden and like a needle through the heart. A hundred times daily. So bittersweet. I hate them, but I love them. I don't want to be without them. I can't live with them. Life is a paradox, for sure. Memories of you... never sitting up to the table bare-chested, even when it was only us. Your back, your neck, your smile, your crooked teeth, your big face, your chest, your hairy chest; your strange, flat, wide, hairless feet; your ears, lobe-less just like mine; your eyelashes, your belly. The feel of your warm body next to mine, your snoring, your snoring while wide awake (!) shaking the bed with my body – a sign for you to turn over. How can I live without all these, and without so much more? For sure I can only write a few, but they are myriad, and I miss you every single day.

Facebook post, 11th October 2015

RANDOM OBSERVATIONS:

1. *There are no swifts in Chania in October. The city is poorer without them.*
2. *In Chania everyone smokes; you even get an ashtray in your room.*
3. *Ten old ladies, in big bathing suits and coloured swimming caps, wade deep into the sea and then float in a circle for hours, talking and laughing, looking for all the world like flotsam and as though this has been a ritual since they were young girls.*
4. *How come, if smoking and sunburn are so bad for you, the world is so full of old, burnt folks smoking?*
5. *I'm at that point in a holiday where you keep seeing folk you think you know. Today I saw HS and JJ and felt lonely because I wanted to say hi!*
6. *English voices, so piercing and annoying and loud…*
7. *There's only one seagull in Chania – I hope she's not lonely.*

Marino Branch
Brainse Marino
Tel: 8336297

And on another day:

Facebook post observations, 12th October 2015

1.   *There are no diving birds; I miss watching the gannets off the coast of Scotland.*
2.   *Let sleeping dogs lie; there are hundreds of them in this small city, just lying around. It seems a good metaphor for my life.*
3.   *Those awkward moments when you realise you're actually drinking from the carafe, or eating straight from the salad bowl? They are the moments you wish you had a pal to hoot with.*
4.   *All the solo travellers all eating in the same place, all adopting the middle-distance stare. Tonight I wanted to gather us all in, as Acorn would say, and have a right knees-up.*
5.   *The more I drink, the more I 'see', the less I can function to write it down.*
6.   *A young man waits every evening in the harbour; he clicks his tongue, he waits patiently, and slowly he gathers cats around him. More arrive. He looks Pied Piperesque as he eventually spreads a feast of cat food, and they dive in, too hungry to growl or spit at one another. It's an unusual sight in a city so unconcerned with animal welfare.*
7.   *Five dark-skinned, bearded, beautiful young*

musicians play their hearts out in a bar where hardly
anyone is paying attention. I do; I am the odd one out.

A brief moment of creativity arrived in the shape of a song. It's only my second song in three years. I grabbed it before it floated away again.

Hey, lady, it's a sore one – there's no playing in me.
The strings of my guitar don't sing and my nails are long
and raggedy.
Hey, mister, you're a strong one and you're stronger than
me.
There's a wind that rocks my soul; I'm lonesome and way
too free.
And all these days are broken and wide, and my heart's
a stranger.
And all the nights are cracked and splintered, and my
soul's in mortal danger.
Hey, my lover, you're a long time gone – it's as hard as
can be.
Through the wandering of my restless days, I am lost to
me.
Because there's a wind that rocks my soul – it's a sirocco,
and it's the lonesome in me.

Monday – different pension:

Diary, 13th October 2015

I'm up with the lark this morning. I am up slightly earlier than required but it means I have the roof terrace all to myself and have secured a front-row seat to watch the sun come up across the harbour, and watch and hear the city come to life. It's beautiful and ancient and warm and I'm feeling very solidly in the world and content. I can't believe it's Monday already! Nearly time to go home. It's been really helpful being here; I feel braver and much more confident. I have been having positive support from pals back home and that has greatly aided my travels.

Facebook post, 13th October 2015

OBSERVATIONS:
1. *Cigarettes are like wee pals; they keep you company when you don't know what to do...*
2. *Travelling solo feels OK; it is pretty safe as long as you watch your back and bag, as you would in any city. The only time I feel freaked out is at the thought of a fall or cutting my feet at the beach or some kind of accident. No one to pick you up and dust you off, and I think the loneliness then would be so overwhelming, coupled with shock, it would be a recipe for a proper breaking down. A big accident would be different –*

services would arrive, folk would administer – but a small fall, a break, a sprain, would be miserable on your own. I tread very carefully.

3. Strangely, being so far away from home has helped me feel connected, much more than when I left. Thanks for your company, Facebookers, and for helping me not go completely mad on my holidays. I've learnt some lessons this week: contact, honesty, community.

4. I'm being very naughty. There are so many people taking photos it's impossible to not end up in them. I'm doing a V-sign on my face or head while being caught in the frame of their cameras.

5. Even though the Victorian carriages and the tired horses are gone from the harbour area, the area still smells strongly of horses. I love that.

Diary, 23rd October 2015

Something has shifted in me. It happened on Jasper's six-month anniversary; I have not written about it but have thought on it a lot since then. There was a physical lifting, as though someone got up from the full length of my body and walked away. It was so profound that I sat up in bed and made a surprised noise, and I could feel the space that had been left behind. At that moment the sun broke through. It was an amazing moment in my journey. It was accompanied by thoughts that I could wake every day for the rest of my life and feel the weight of my loss. I was mulling over how much of my burden

I could lay down. I believe it was a powerful healing moment for me. It bizarrely and neatly bookends both of us falling into despair three years ago as we realised Jasper was proper poorly, and my six months of widowhood. This all happened before I went to Crete, but it definitely helped me to be strong enough to get on the plane and get there.

Winter 2015/16

Since coming back from Chania a week ago I have felt much more confident and able to be sociable, and also to be alone a bit more. The flat is beginning to feel more like home, and I have nearly finished unpacking. So strange to find how much I gave away or threw out when I had to move suddenly in May. Jasper would be proud of my lack of stuff. (There's still loads, though not too much.)

Diary, 29th October 2015

Here I be, back on our beloved isle and in the company of Donald, Heather and Dolphin Boy for five days. House-sitting for friends, in a gorgeous new build, light and airy, warm and cosy, so much space. I woke today to the sound of the rain and the birds.

Yesterday was very special. I don't know if I can convey it here, but I will try. A gorgeous drive up from Edinburgh via Dalwhinnie through the breaking dawn. When we arrived at the port, we discovered the Lochnevis (big boat) was broken and instead we were travelling by a tiny thirty-four-person catamaran. The incredible thing about our crossing was that we were accompanied, a good part of the way, by over two hundred dolphins! Two hundred! Two hundred!!! Oh my, a once-in-a-lifetime sight; it was as though the sea was boiling. They swan alongside, under and behind our boat. They surfed the bow waves. Everywhere you looked there were dolphins. I never thought I would see such a sight. I have longed all my days to see just one! Ha! It helped shift the gentle numbness that has descended and now sits over my heart. I'm not feeling much again and Jasper is hard to locate. My mind and heart slide away from getting too close to flashbacks and memory. It pulls me back from the point of engagement and the point of pain. I hope it's just a phase. I am afraid now of losing the ability to locate Jasper in my mind and my heart. But almost in the same breath I can say I see him more clearly as he really was, not my 'telephone guy' but my actual guy. He is just there in my head, all the time, a part of me always. So, I know he would have hated this little boat, he would have enjoyed the dolphins a little bit, but he would have enjoyed my excitement a lot. I miss you.

Our tiny boat docked but the tide was so low we had to disembark onto a set of very slimy stairs, covered in barnacles and seaweed. I was so glad to spot a pair of

*yellow wellies and a strong arm and I knew that Dean
was there, one arm firmly anchored around a seaweed-
covered post, the other reaching over to help folks get from
the boat, across the boiling sea onto the slippy steps. In
my heart I was very glad, because if anyone slipped and
went in the sea, I knew he would not hesitate to try and
save them.*

Diary, 30th October 2015

*Today I hope to play music with Donald and sing a few
songs and be in the world.*

*Dreams of Jasper shady and indistinct. It's not just
that you died and that you are gone from my physical
life, and how shocking that is to try and assimilate. It's the
three years of sorrow and stress and fear, and then finally
the last six to eight months of darkness that came before
you died, the loss of you as the person you had always
been. October 2014 to April 2015 were a horror. A pure
horror. We held on as best we could, my love, we held true,
but Lordy, we were cracking and splintering right enough,
and who could have done any better with such a strain?
You watched me break my heart, over and over, for the
losing of you, and I watched your heart and mind break
along with your poor, sweet, sore body. Oh, my love, what
things we saw, what pain you carried. It's nearly seven
months since your pain ended, and I am grateful you are
no longer in pain. I feel low today; less alcohol will help,
and some time on my own. I am practising keeping quiet
when perturbed or annoyed, and it's working better for*

me. I miss you, Jasper; I keep seeing you walking along the road. I know how much you would have loved being here on the island with our friends. You always loved this house. Tonight, I am wondering – what is the colour of my heart? The world has come down to who I feel safe with. There are a number of people, and I seek them out. They are the folks who will not feel uncomfortable if I'm blue, who will let me speak your name, and laugh with me as we remember you. They have no idea how much I value them, how much I need them in my life. I try not to be a burden; I try not to be needy. I try to be 'fun'. They see through me sometimes and hold me close. Your best friend Dave is the person I like to spend time with the most. We talk and talk and talk about you. We grieve and laugh together, and it feels so good. So safe. He was a good choice, my love. He is a good friend to me now. You would be so very proud of him.

Grief seekers. I had never heard this term before I became a carer for my terminally ill husband. I laughed out loud when a friend first mentioned she had been reading about them in a book. She advised me to take care, to steer clear of such people. I laughed because I just couldn't believe this type of people really existed. If only I had been right. They do, and they will stop at nothing to make sure you know that their pain is as strong and deep for your loved one as yours. *Your* pain – the pain you yourself can't even begin to articulate, the pain of a shattered life, of the loss of your best friend, your lover, the father to your child, the person you have shared every aspect of your life with. This makes no sense to me. Why would someone want to feel this bad?

I had many emails and Facebook messages over the time

Jasper was ill, and after his death, from kind people meaning well, and I don't ever regret reading those messages, although they were upsetting at times. However, I truly objected to one person, whom I have never met, and who had not been in my husband's life for over thirty years (and then only briefly as a friend for one short summer). She wrote me many times after she heard about him being ill through a mutual old friend, expressing how terrible she was feeling about his illness, how she couldn't cope with the prospect of his loss. It utterly terrified and bewildered me, this imposter in our lives who thought she had the right, and the depth of love for my husband. In the end, I asked him to contact her and tell her it was too much. He and I even had cross words about it, so keen was he to not make a fuss, to protect her from my lack of ability, and the lack of my availability, to absorb her 'grief'. It had been so long since they had been in touch she even called him by a name I had never heard him use. It was astonishing to me, this woman's lack of care for how I would feel having to deal with her inappropriate contact. So strange to receive an email talking about some bloke I had never met, didn't know, some bloke with another name...

There were others – a young man who had had an affair with a friend's wife, and the affair had ended badly after only a matter of weeks. He wanted to talk to me about how our 'situations' were just the same. I was stumped by this and anxiously mumbled, "Yes, yes, of course, loss is loss", while all the time thinking, *How can this be the same? How can eighteen years of commitment be the same as a few short weeks of an affair? And she is still alive; you still have* hope *that you may work things out. I have* no *hope. My time with my husband is over. It can never be reclaimed or rekindled.* How very strange.

Hi, you don't know me but...
Hello, I hope this doesn't upset you...

I recently received a Facebook message from a woman I have never met, but who is 'following' me on Facebook (such a strange term – don't follow me, I am lost...). She messaged me several times saying she had a message from Jasper for me and would I want to hear it? I ignored this, as I tend to do. Simply not responding is quite often enough of a deterrent. However, she was very persistent, and in her fourth email, while acknowledging I had not responded to her, so maybe I simply didn't want to know, she told me she had been walking in the woods, trying to remember his name, and suddenly she remembered and said it aloud and he appeared in her thoughts saying, *That's my name, don't wear it out!* and grinning hugely. She said he had asked her to pass along a message: he was with me, he loved me, it was hard to see me struggle, and he liked my new glasses. (The glasses bit was the only part that I felt resonated even slightly.)

It's not that I don't believe he is somewhere, probably quite nearby, but I find it hard to fathom why he would talk to someone we both don't know, someone who lives thousands of miles away, to get such a simple message to me. I know he loves me; I know he is close. But if he is, why isn't he giving me a hard time about smoking again after twelve years of not doing... why wouldn't he say something only we could recognise as ours? I didn't reply to her.

By November 2015 I'm panicking. I don't sleep for more than two hours at a stretch; I'm anxious, very lonely and so bone-tired. I go to sleep OK but wake full of terror. Am I dead? Where am I? What's gone wrong? Where are you? I no longer cry at all; instead my grief is like a dead weight that takes all my air and causes such inertia. I am profoundly depressed and isolated. I spend the hours between 1am and 6.30am reading and ruminating. All the things I could have done differently. All the things I should have done differently. I'm scared of sleeping pills – what if I can't wake from the night terrors that torment me?

Christmas is looming. The shops are a minefield. The question on shopkeepers' lips – "Are you looking forward to Christmas?" *No!* I am dreading it. You loved Christmas. You made it fun. You're not here. It's my first without you. I have planned to be away from Edinburgh; to travel south and be with the folks who knew you best. My two-week trip involves lots of social time, lots of different houses. How will I cope? I will spend the majority of it with Dave and Marion. I'm looking forward to being in company. To piggybacking on other people's lives. To being amongst our friends. Anything will be better than this awful loneliness. Our city is not my city any more. I think about suicide every day now. I am deeply worried about me.

I decide to rent the flat out on Airbnb while I'm away. I totally mess up the registration, a sign I'm not ready. I find myself inundated with bookings through December and into the New Year. Damn. This means I must pack away my personal possessions, clean the flat repeatedly, meet strangers, show them around my home, and clear out elsewhere while they are here. What have I done? It's too much for me, and I realise I really am not fit enough mentally to take the added strain. It's too late, though. It's all confirmed. I somehow get through this awful month of November and find, when I begin writing this memoir, a bit of peace, but it also puts me right back into the dreadful times we went through. I'm shocked at how much I have blanked out, and how little physical evidence there is of our times. Remembering brings such bittersweet emotions, and another series of nightmares.

Diary, 4th December 2015

What will become of me? I feel so hopeless, lonely, and as though there's no place for me any more. I am horribly insecure. I miss you, my love. I can't wait to join you – yes, I did just write that. I just can't see a way through my life without you here to hold my hand. To sit with me, to be my friend.

I head south on 24th December. It feels so good to leave the city, and when I arrive at Dave and Marion's I'm immediately scooped up and cared for. I can breathe again. I have made the right decision. I spend two weeks cruising around, visiting friends, being back in the world, and find my anxiety has largely disappeared; I'm even sleeping better and I can be sociable. I can have fun. It's real. Dave and I spend a few nights sitting up all night, drinking whisky, talking about you, remembering, enjoying our times, crying and laughing. It feels so good. My heart and soul feel as though they are filling up again. Maybe I am not so lost after all.

Dave and Marion invite me to come live with them. It's unbelievable how good and safe this makes me feel. I don't think I will, but to be asked, for it to be recognised that I am not coping, that my grief needs to be cared for, is immense. It changes things for me. I head back to Edinburgh feeling better than I have for over three years. I have survived 2015. I will keep going. And most importantly, I realise – I really do want to live.

I understand that I need to be in company, to spend time with people. If I'm on my own too much the world caves in and I become profoundly depressed. This can come over me in the course of only a few hours, and so I begin to look after myself better. I begin to value myself again. I knock the solo drinking on the head (mostly), I give up the fags (again, mostly) and I begin a programme of swimming and walking every day. I'm back to four juices, most days, and healthy eating. This all feeds into a much healthier mindset. I decide I want a future, and that future will be a house built on our beloved island. To that end I try to apply for permission to build on a vacant plot.

Somewhere in there I decide to try to take tamoxifen again. I take advice from Maggie's Centre and my oncology consultant and, yes, it's still a 'good idea' as it will offer protection against recurrence. Five days into it I'm on the floor with nausea and toxicity. I pull back. I consider the cannabis oil. I still have two full treatments. They are my safety. I have no idea how long they will keep for.

Diary, 17th January 2016

Today became one of those days, those missing-you days, where I'm fine and then suddenly I'm not. I changed from a coping widow to a mess in a matter of minutes. I fell into pure missing of that man. Not a peripheral, Where are you, husband? but deep into the nitty-gritty of your missing self. The absolute, simple, everyday faces and motions and saying and ways that made you, you. I miss those, those teeny-tiny ways, your care, your essence and what that meant to me. Grief is so subjective; this is what makes it so hard to convey. I miss a different Jasper than others do. That's a lonely place. You were the only one I had that relationship with. Other folk had a different one. We can all talk about you and, yes, there is a myriad of common ground, stuff that is universal. I put Billy Bragg on the car stereo and suddenly there you were, standing in our old living room in our early days of courting, grinning at me, and singing along to New England at full tilt. Such strong memories. I broke down at the traffic lights, tears on the Southside; my broken heart rose out of me and swamped me. It caught me. I see you.

I got lost in my grief, but, importantly, back at the new flat, I called out for help. I rang Dave and I rang Acorn, and we talked and cried and laughed, and they helped me pull back from the edge again.

Facebook post, 24th February 2016

Save the date – 3rd April 2016.

Hi, pals; folks have been asking what I might do for Jasper's first anniversary. It's a bit odd as there are two dates: Good Friday is on 24th March this coming year, and the actual anniversary date of his passing is 3rd April.

I will head south for Good Friday and be with Dave and Marion in their home where we spent many silly and happy times.

For Sunday 3rd April I would love to meet some, any, all of you, everyone welcome, at 3pm in the car park at the observatory and take a stroll around Blackford Hill. If the weather's warm enough, as it was last year, we could stop for a while at the bit overlooking Midmar and the west coast. Sit, look, huddle, eat some picnic, maybe even play some tunes and chuck some balls in the air. Dave and Marion will be with us too, I think/I hope. It may be that we can also share some memories of Jasper and raise a glass to him? I may even bring his big, yellow, smiley flag and raise it, so I can remember that beautiful smile and how chuffed he was when I gifted the flag to him. This is all weather dependent – but hopefully the sun will shine and we can at least get out for a walk. Later on, I'm going to head down to Bells Diner for dinner at 7pm – if you're up for this, please phone and book your own table. If things progress we may even end up back at my flat for a bit of a nightcap.

I know you won't be able to be with us, Sue Collins, as you will probably be mid-air en route back from Oz. It didn't seem right not to include you, and, as we had such a profound and 'state of grace' time on Blackford Hill last year on that weekend, I know you will be able to picture us very clearly and raise a glass to Jasper, if that fits.

I like the above plan. I hope you can join in.

Lots of love, Sharon.

(Yes, I know, I am way ahead with planning, as usual. Funny, though; planning this coming year's anniversary is helping me through the nightmare year I'm currently in.)

Facebook post, 3rd April 2016

Today marks a year since Jasper passed away. I truly still can't believe that he's not here and that a year has gone by. But somehow it has.

The loneliness and isolation without him keeping me right, and us laughing together, have been at times unbearable, despite everyone's best efforts. It was always going to be so. There is an agoraphobia in grief, with so many spaces that are Jasper-shaped. For the ongoing support from family, friends and Maggie's Centre, and for sticking with me through the madness and depression that this year has brought, always my deepest gratitude.

I've been countering some of the memories of days in hospice and our grief, with better memories of our happiest times: with Jasper in great form on Eigg; handsome, strong and funny; the way he should be remembered. It's been a bittersweet delight to see him in our home movies, and to see him again so clearly. I have been lost in days and nights of editing on the clunky, rubbish Windows Movie Maker program, while the computer groaned and crashed and couldn't keep up. It's been comfortingly slow. I hope it doesn't seem indulgent to have used the gig video; it's all I have for footage and we are having fun. I've pondered a lot about posting it. I hope you don't mind. I hope the people who loved him find comfort in it, and that it makes you smile.

The video is a few wee snippets of one day on Eigg and our meanderings, and of our first ever scratch gig as Mr and Mrs King, on a summer evening in 2011, playing for our supper. There's a whole lot of love in the Lageorna room; we are a bit ropy gig-wise, but we are loving playing together. It was very hard to edit it down to these ten minutes.

I'm going into the Marie Curie hospice at Liberton today to make a donation. I've also set up a JustGiving memorial page for Jasper; the money donated will be used in Marie Curie hospices to help others with end-of-life care.

Please raise a cup of tea, as Jasper would have done, today around 1pm, to a beautiful soul and a shining light; a one-in-a-million husband, my best friend, a Harry Handsome disco dancer, a man of steel, a world traveller. Juggler and balancer extraordinaire, a comic, a clown and a musician; Jasper Chipolata. Jasper was a loving son and stepson, brother and stepbrother, and a brilliant stepdad, a total family man. He was an avid Liverpool supporter and crazy about golf, competitive and pretty talented at most things, excepting pushbikes, horses and DIY. Jasper was a gentle and loving man, one of a kind; he is missed by so many, always in my head and in my heart. Words aren't enough. I feel him in the sunshine and he walks beside me every day. x

December 2016 to April 2017

I've not read anything that has come before this in an attempt to not get pulled back in there. On the advice of my psychologist at Maggie's I started taking the antidepressant citalopram in the lead-up to Jasper's first anniversary. They floored me at first, I was so tired I was eyeing up the ground in supermarkets and street doorways, wishing only that I could just lie down. I would nod off everywhere and driving was tricky, especially on long journeys. I had to keep pulling off the road to sleep in my seat until I could drive again. It was a vast, deep tiredness that could not be denied. It was the true exhaustion that comes once the cortisol, which has been running on fight or flight for years, begins to recede; however this recession can take a very long time. Cortisol is the body's main stress hormone and is made by the adrenal glands; it controls mood, fear and motivation. I think of suicide every day now but I know I won't do it; how could I possibly cause more pain to my friends and family? How could I leave my parents to manage alone into their old age, how could I deny my daughter a grandmother for her future children and my loving presence? My Maggie's therapist tells me it's normal to have these thoughts, they are only a safety mechanism; by considering my own death I have a way to feel I have a choice. I am afraid, though, and at times the pull is so strong. I think of the ways I can do it so it looks like an accident, so I won't be held accountable. I think I am losing the will to keep going. The fear is so strong it's like a tide that washes over me, mostly late at night, when I am alone. I can't tell these thoughts to anyone apart from my Maggie's lady. Who could understand this? It feels overly dramatic and attention-seeking, and I feel ashamed for even considering it. And so the downward spiral spins…

However, the pills have allowed a lot of the panic and fear to recede; a thin veil hangs over my grief and that has allowed light to enter again. It's allowed me some respite from rumination and given me confidence to manage daily tasks. The very large downside is a lack of creativity, zilch. I have shied away from beginning to write again because I now live in a place where I don't examine and fret; it's a fairly stress-free place, a huge relief, and I'm much better socially for it. Dark days still come, but they don't feel so dangerous and though I mull over leaving this life, I don't feel drawn to it. It has become an abstract thought again and continues to be a bit of a safety valve.

I spent this summer in the caravan again. It was much easier than last year, but still very lonely and I managed to fall on the beach, after much whisky-drinking, and break my right wrist. It took me two weeks to leave the island to go and have it x-rayed, and I returned to Eigg in a plaster cast. I can't quite believe I worked two weeks chambermaiding with a broken wrist. I am amazed at my stupidity and my intensely high level of pain tolerance.

I've been busy setting up and raising funds for a new trust me, Rani and some friends are forming in Jasper's name. The money raised will enable folks affected by a cancer diagnosis to holiday on the island for seven days at a time. We are doing very well with our fundraising and 2017 holidays have been booked in and paid for. The trust is being formalised with our lawyers (how posh does that sound? I've never had a lawyer in my life), and we should be a registered charity by end of June 2017.

I have decided next summer I will have just one month in the caravan and be there while our trust visitors are holidaying, to help them with any questions or problems that may arise. The caravan is all I have left of our old life together and I relish its presence and opportunity for escape in my life. I silently give thanks to Wes and Maggie every day for allowing me to have this space on the croft. I still dream of a house on Eigg, but I know it will never be a new build. I am very poor and could never manage such a huge undertaking on my own.

It's funny; I used to feel Jasper in the sun, but these days more and more I feel he is in the zephyrs and the breezes, and I walk and wander and think of him. I am glad our journey is bringing some small comfort to others who access the funding to holiday on the island. The small comforts mean a lot to me. I wonder what Jasper would think of it all. I suspect he would throw his head back and laugh heartily at the absurdity of it.

I've moved again. Suzys flat now feels too far out of the main part of the city and I have grieved so deeply there, it seems to come back out of the walls at me. I am renting a friend's flat in Leith, just off the Walk, top floor, open fire, lovely Victorian flat with a large, sunny office/bedroom. I keep waiting for the catch. I love it and feel very much at home. I can feel myself emerging further out into the world of dinners and pubs and people. I'm hoping creativity may arrive soon...

It's so much easier to be alone these days – have I just got used to it? There are now many aspects I enjoy when I am solitary. I am beginning college in September, studying for an HND in travel and tourism. Why? It's just a way to get out of the house, to get a student loan so I can survive financially, and possibly in the future to enable me to begin again with a new career. But my heart's not in it; I simply attend, do the work and get through the days. However, attending college has also thrown up a reason for a lifetime of difficulties I have experienced in processing information and in repeatedly falling over, especially when I am stressed. I have been tested by an educational psychologist and I now have a certificate; I have a condition called dyspraxia, which is a relation to dyslexia, another information processing condition. Dyspraxia causes problems with spatial awareness and general clumsiness and explains so much. It is a relief to have a reason for the many falls and poor short-term memory function, which I have always struggled with.

I find myself busy enough to not feel so lonely when I'm alone. I drink far too much and have taken up smoking pretty much full time. My body is in very poor shape and I'm due at the breast clinic on Thursday for a lung CT. My right breast and chest wall are causing me a lot of pain, I cannot turn over in bed, and rising from sitting or lying down is agony. The antidepressants allow me to be largely unconcerned, and that also is the rub… I ponder a lot on what happens after life and if I will somehow find my energy caught up with his as we spin in the winds.

I perform my first gig in over three years and manage to give a very good account of myself. Two more gigs booked for the end of February and beginning of March. I can't see further than that for music. The energy just may not be there. I am in the world again, but I am exhausted by it. I enjoy hiding now for a few days at a time. It feels so good to be able to be alone. My phone is off; I am pottering and sleeping and just being sat sitted. I think of Jasper a lot, countless times every day. Some days he is very close, and they are hard days. Other days it's as if I was never in my previous life. The past twenty years seem like a dream. I feel so very changed. I have been burnt through a fire of hell and loss, and the 'me' I am now is not the 'me' I was before 2013.

I take cannabis oil, a tiny amount every day, along with prescribed exemestane, an avuncular therapy for breast cancer prevention. I have been prescribed this in the hope I will tolerate it better than the tamoxifen. I have no idea where my body and mind will take me next. I have lost my way with the organic alkalising diet but feel I have found some strength in my soul to keep trying to live in the world, and I hope the healthy approach will come back to me in time.

Diary, 9th March 2017

So strange to be so adept at pretending to be in the world; chat, chat, chat – and to feel so removed. Is this how it will be? Is this what people do?

I am aware of an increasing realisation: it's changing again; I am becoming more physical, and wouldn't it be so good to have a pal, a cuddling, sexual pal to have adventures with? To go to festivals, dress up, act like idiots, laugh and cuddle and lay in the sun. I want this more and more, just a pal to make plans with. How do you do that? I don't want any more than that, but I am all at sea in the courting game. I don't leave the house or socialise with people who aren't old friends or couples; no singles there. Do I advertise? No, I am not ready – I am lonely, but prefer my own company and I think I am too afraid of someone seeing the darkness in my soul and heart, and ultimately of being rejected or hurt.

Diary, 13th March 2017

I can feel the Black Dog circling; he is still at a distance, enough that if I choose I could make some calls, ask for some support over the next few weeks. Pride, stupid pride, but also I know I crave solitude – how to marry the need to be held and the need to hide? Business is the key, but that requires energy and planning; two things the Black Dog takes away. At least I am learning what a slide into depression feels like. Is it so simple as to let folks know I am struggling? They say they want to know, but do they really? My eternal fight with myself when the dog is around; by the time he is on my chest I will be too far in it to reach out. It has to be now…

The weeks leading up to significant dates are often worse than the day itself. The dreaded day has a purpose. It's here; the hours go by at whatever pace; the dying and funeral hours were deeply traumatic last year. I fear for the days ahead. Roll on May.

I managed to reach out; I sent a text to several people, simply asking them to keep me in mind and send me a bit of love and strength. God, it's so hard to admit I'm not coping! I had a great response and I am feeling held, and the voice in my head that mocks me, telling me I am alone and worthless, has receded again.

Onset of depression – the signs: feeling isolated, no energy, rumination, insomnia, fear of the future, fear of outside, social anxiety, muddled thinking, weeping, inability to make decisions, lack of appetite and care for myself, compulsive behaviour, spending too much money, thoughts of death, irritation with people and the 'small problems'.

Spring is here; I have the bedroom window open this morning. A winter without snow, a better one for me than last year; looking back it's clear to see I am coping much better with life; grief lives more like a shadow and less like a knife. I can find peace in my solitude and I can believe in a future.

By 31st March 2017 I have nearly finished the Whole30 programme; no alcohol for twenty-six days and I feel as though I have some control back in my life for the first time in many years.

I have come off the exemestane breast cancer medication. It was causing dreadful, chronic pain in my chest wall and ribs, and is possibly the reason for my two new broken ribs which happened spontaneously in the late autumn of 2016. Along with feeling better physically I also have clarity of thinking which has been absent for a very long time, part grief, part exemestane, I suspect. I don't think I will be going back on the medication. I will take my chances and be healthy while I'm healthy. What's the point in taking a drug that makes you so ill you can't function in the world? And it's a world I'm keener to be involved in these days.

Diary, 3rd April 2017 – your second anniversary

'It's Time'
Time is a tyrant; no limits, no naughty step, no time out.
Marching and stretching, bending and doubling back on
*   itself; a tangled ball.*
Time is a generous giver, if unexpected.
Gifting endless days for good or for bad.

Time is a heartbeat, a handclap, a foot stomp, a da da da.

Time, WTF?

Time is as old as... time, and as young as the future, unless already visited...

On an untimely trip, an Escher staircase, a waiting room.

Time needs filled, but time is not empty.

Time heals? Time numbs, distorts, distracts, contracts,

Creates difference and forward motion.

Time doesn't give a shit about healing.

Time is only time.

Diary, 9th April 2017

Where would you be just now, Jasper, if our situations had been reversed? I can't imagine. I don't want to imagine you lonely and self-conscious, a bit agoraphobic. It's been two years since I have been held; longer, really. I reckon more like four or five years in terms of sexual intimacy. Yes, we had intimacy in the latter years, but it was so different, like parent and child, or brother and sister; deep love, deep and enduring love, but not like we were. I want to feel excited by connections, to daydream and create amazing real-life days, new times, memories that aren't overlaid with grief. Is this wrong of me? How long, how long...?

When your heart pulls – drawn in by an invisible thread and ink (black), and the rules of the universe are splintered and don't apply, and endless days go; by, by, bye.

And long-time friends don't know where to look, where is the book? Unwritten, but already a bestseller.

My fella, the one, the world, here I am profoundly undone. It is so lonely here and most times I have lost your face, your voice, your smell.

Diary, 15th April 2017

Yesterday's funeral anniversary spent in Bradford with Dave, Marion and old friends. A lovely picnic lunch round the kitchen table, wine and singing 'I'll Fly Away', and then to the park to fly kites, but there was no wind. We had lots of laughs and whisky and toasts to you. My heart feels easier today. I just needed company, people to be with who knew you well. Another reminder of how lonely Edinburgh is for me.

May to December 2017

Diary, 15th May 2017

Words; I never thought that words would become an enemy. To write with clarity and flow yields beauty and understanding, a view that is universal, but to read, edit, delve deeper into those words can be traumatic and so, and maybe this is key, I have lost my words, because I am scared of what I may say. We all live in the bubble, all looking in at ourselves and each other... judgements and denials. I live now in denial, in an accepting kind of way, if that can make sense. I live alone, I live in my past; the two don't meet, but I try to reconcile them. I fail. I have not written for so long; again, because words, if I write them down, will bite me. But there is laziness there also. I just can't be arsed. I keep asking myself the question, do I really care, does it matter, how long can I keep this up?

Will he be waiting for me, if I die? Is there more? I am curious, but no longer dangerously so. How long can

I live in a world that I do not believe in? Is this just part of the 'process'?

I was gifted a week at Harvest Moon; I spent it laughing with old pals, roaming the beach, roaring with the wind. Soul-filled times.

Diary, 23rd May 2017, Sloan Street

I have been listening to Emmylou singing 'Goodbye' and I am transported back to the crematorium and all the questions that will never be answered. These tie into my rumination that we never actually got to say goodbye. I came back to the hospice after a long afternoon at the flat, dealing with the estate agent and then sitting in our sunny window in exhaustion and disbelief. I was losing you; our life together was fading; our rented home of ten years was being sold. I had been told by the doctor at the hospice, you only had weeks left. I was hollow with burnout and dread.

I returned to find you in agony and you looked at me and said, "Where the fuck have you been?"; so unlike you and I am so sorry. I fumbled a reply about chores and shopping. I lied to you because I couldn't bear to tell you the truth. I could not burden you further, even though it meant absorbing your anger and fear. You never knew what had happened at home that day, and I am thankful. I will take that, for all the world. For sure.

And then, the next day, they put you under, like we always thought they would, but I didn't believe it, I thought there would be more time, another chance to hold you and tell you how much I loved you. I brushed off your attempts to say goodbye. I couldn't bear to hear it. You died two days later.

Diary, 16th June 2017

College finished yesterday. I did it; I got through this academic year. It's been really tough going at times, particularly with the lead-up to end of term; I lost my focus and for a while it looked as if I would not make it through. I start again in August. In the meantime I will return to Eigg and the caravan for a while to see the Jasper King Trust families through their holidays. I am terrified to return to the caravan. It has become a terribly lonely place for me, a place I have grieved and gone mad in.

I am lying in bed, enjoying the prospect of a 'no-do day'. I am just back from Eden Festival – six days and nights in the tiny tent and the pouring rain. I have been working for my ticket with the Melodrome Crew; Mick and Michele invited me when they heard me say I have no forward motion, no invites because I have turned down too many. Bless them for taking action on my behalf. I did really well, compèring, singing, washing dishes. I got it, they got it. I spent a lot of time hiding in my tent, writing, thinking, re-energising. But I was in the world, I was a person doing normal things, making conversations with people I don't know, and this is a big step forward.

Diary, 20th June 2017 (Midsummer)

Long, hot days, time spent in street cafes...

I am reflecting back on Saturday's dog-day afternoon – in spite of the sunshine, or because? In spite of the cool local vibe at the Elvis Shakespeare book and record shop; crowd clapping, sun beaming, musicians playing... I left. I stomped home, prepared for and on the threshold of a why/what/when session, and there on my doorstep was a gift of sea-glass jewellery and no note. The mystery of the gift caused the Black Dog to settle nearby; not on my chest as he had planned, and while he whispered, Whisky and wine – you'll be fine, I enjoyed the mystery of who had sent such a special gift. It also put me in mind of the many kindnesses shown over the years; messages, gifts, time spent and kind words, and how small acts of kindness really did help my feelings of being lost or forgotten.

Strange days, drifting, quiet, not much contact; when there is I am random, stoned, a bit daft, hiding, hiding, hiding. It's exhausting. I have got so good at hiding I don't know how to be any other way with people. Is this it? Is this all there will be from now on? I feel I am slowly fading from the world; my points of reference are not part of the world view of the people I interact with. Many days I don't speak apart from to say, "Green tea, please" and "Thank you, bus driver." I am losing the will to try socially. I am getting worse. I am getting concerned for myself again.

Exquisite Torture

Woken from slumber – a long, bereaved sleep – by a vital spark that rolled, then leapt between us.

A long weekend, planned with only an old friend, became an insane and exquisite torture.

Clichéd lightning bolts, electrical currents, longing sublime, shocking. Overwhelming restraint;

We walked a fine, fine line through honesty and sexual tension. Hold the line. Hold. Holding allowed, but no kissing, not much sleeping.

Waves of desire fuelled by the fire of long-time loneliness. A perfect storm;

A beautiful, handsome pal, trust, connection, deep loneliness and a need for attention,

Driven not by one but by the two of us. Both in a world of isolation and alienation, both starved of affection. Oh, what an exquisite torture!

Two nights sharing beds, but holding the line with cuddles and a lot of soul-searching.

Eyes on eyes. And time stopping; the feeling in our bodies, outrageous and shocking;

Intensity, ferocity, coming alive and vibrating, and the line creating an exquisite delight.

Hold the line; a battle raging, instinct pushing for a resolution. Kiss him, kiss him – no, hold the line; exhausting.

Talking and talking, talking of our lives and realising the horror of knowing; this is the madness of falling. We are broken. Hold the line.

A long drive home to say goodbye to a weekend, unintended, that has shattered the sky.

No touching, scared to meet eyes, lightning bolts and truth and the pain of goodbye.

Resolution; no contact, no alone, no texts, no phone.

Diary, 6th July 2017

Huge changes of late; I feel scrubbed, sand-blown by a warm sirocco. Life has moved on so fast in the past two weeks and I am not processing, just revelling in the tide of hope, desire, future fun. I have been having fun this past while just being out in the world. So unexpected, so overwhelming; how can things change so fast – do I now want to, really want to live again? Yes, I think I do.

Festivals are hard work; I'm tired and broken but I am alive! I am interested, mostly, and can play the game; say the right thing, appear normal, have fun, be funny, be me, or go to bed for twelve hours, hide in my tent, listen to the radio, miss Jasper but feel confident in myself, in my solitude. I must remember that the beer goggles lie and I must remember I am still lonely, still vulnerable. On Saturday I am meeting this person who has awakened me; we are going to lunch. What will it be like? I hope it's not as powerful. I am scared of my desire; I am scared of doing a bad thing. I need to be patient. Go steady, my love, I hear Jasper whisper. I hear you, husband.

Diary, 23rd July 2017

A beautiful, silent, soul-filled day of sunshine and pottering at the caravan. Finally, a feeling of contented peace; happy to just be, sitting in the sun, swinging in the hammock, meditating on life and just being.

Hello to Eigg!

*Hello to Eigg, the jewel in the crown of the islands that
halo the west coast of Scotland.*

*Hello to the pier, the hellos and "How long are you
here?"*

*Hello to the boys, the caravan crew, the 'Gaza Strip'
team: me, Shuggy and Dean.*

*Hello to the 'Sharavan', somehow still intact, another
winter fared and another year past. Old maid of
a van, my forty-year-old madam, my shelter, my
home, my memories, my deep grieving place.*

*Hello to the new bridge that spans the stream; how I
have longed for you to appear in years past as I
brokenly jumped, sometimes falling in…*

*Hello, Laig Bay, wondrous views and silver sands that
meet your long and rolling waves.*

*Hello to my toes and the shallow-water wading, Atlantic
Ocean rippling in the hot sun and warm zephyrs
playing.*

*Hello, small birds that I live amongst, in my green
gloaming bubble fish tank. I sit and listen and
watch you chatter, through tree- and light-filtered
haze.*

*Hello to the rarefied air and the constant changing
weather, to the highs and the lows and the
disappearing Rum and Sgurr.*

*Hello to the Singing Sands, Shell Beach, and all your
undiscovered treasures. I walk and I walk and still
don't uncover.*

Hello, wild orchids, clear water burn, bracken and
*   heather, bog weed and rushes, sea eagle and*
*   meadow larks.*
Hello to the ceilidh, always one somewhere; hello to the
*   lift home and the care and torch chat.*
Hello to Eigg, the jewel in the crown.

Diary, 2nd August 2017, Edinburgh

I am so glad to be back home. I have had big thoughts
while I was away on Eigg. I acknowledge I can't do this
alone; I don't want to be alone. Nothing ever happens
'cause I'm too busy coping with just being. I want a pal, a
companion, good sex, laughter, dressing up for dates, going
places, just being. Washing the fucking dishes together!
Just being. There is still a long road ahead. The love that
flared in June has died and I am deeply sad. But I am
also pragmatic. I was a fool to think it was anything but a
dream born of two people's loneliness, but, as my daughter
wisely pointed out, from it I learnt I can feel, I can want to
be with someone, and that's worth its weight in gold.

So strange to kiss someone else; it's been eighteen years
of loving one man. His shape is not my husband's shape;
with my eyes closed I felt his body but my body kept telling
me, This is the wrong body. This is the wrong shape. There
is still a long road ahead.

Diary, 17th August 2017, Edinburgh

I feel I am reclaiming parts of myself that have disappeared, they are returning; made brand new by the fire, bit by bit, month by month, year by year. Tonight I played a self-assured gig, five minutes from my front door. I felt local. I am local, and I have the knowledge that this gentle day, slowly getting ready for a gig; this could be life. I can do this.

Language learning

After you died…
We became I,
Us became me,
These is this,
Ours is now mine.

I must be getting better; I now think much more often in the latter terms, and for so long that was very weird. I would constantly be correcting myself: *Ourselves, we, us, ours.*

Diary, 29th September 2017

More changes… my GP has upped my dose of antidepressants. Turns out I've been on the dose for anxiety (ten milligrams), and I really need to be on the dose for depression (between twenty and forty milligrams) – I wish I had known that before now. What a change; energy has returned, I have clarity of thinking, I am capable of excitement and forward motion. I have been so numb and so depressed. I can see it clearly now.

The End and the Beginning

Diary, 26th December 2017

I woke today slightly less hung-over than previous days, after disturbing, strange dreams of monsters and a written piece that must stay hidden. Through my slow morning of musings I realised. I must finish this. I must be done.

And so I set to it, my head filled with images of panic and pain and hospice. In retrospect it's obvious: Boxing Day 2015 was the day we first saw the beginning of the end. I managed two hours of solid writing and organised chapters that had previously defeated me. I feel it's my only way forward, to finish. I see that now. Please, Black Dog, allow me some peace and energy to complete, for good or bad. It may remain only a monument to my grief, to the journey, the process, that I will most probably never read. Or it may become a book which might help someone on a similar journey. Whatever. I have begun again.

May 2018

I am too used to living alone and my solitude. I can't imagine now sharing a house, a bed, a life, always being a part of someone else.

I am strong physically; no broken ribs for over a year – quite an achievement. No return of breast cancer; another achievement.

I drink too much, as always, but I know, and these diary entries are testament, it cannot continue.

Some days are so dark I don't get out of bed. I distract myself with wine and Netflix. I get through it. I know now to courie in and await the return of the life force and the will to eat and live and be, even if it's only marginally.

I am awaiting womb-lining biopsies; mine are way too thick. I try not to worry; I stay in the present. Cancer has taken enough of my time, and taken my true love. I will not dwell on what may not be.

I am a different being wholly from who I was; I am much more level (pills), and I am kinder (compassion). I am patient, no longer a patient. I know it's not all about me.

Although I am chronically and profoundly depressed there are days which are lighter. I despair of life ever being fulfilling. I go to college; I try to be 'normal'. I do the work, but really I don't care; I expect to fail my course, but it doesn't matter. It's the journey, not the arrival.

June 2018

I decided I would finally get a puppy, someone to love and cherish and who would love me unconditionally. I bought a female dog of uncertain parentage from some dodgy people in Haddington; I broke all the 'buying a dog' rules. I didn't care; I just needed her with me, that day, not a day later. I call her Frida Kahlo. She has lightened up my world; she requires attention and feeding and walking and love. She gives so much love in return I don't know, writing this a month later, how I ever lived without her. I couldn't have brought her into my life any earlier, but she is a balm to my depression, and she is a great cuddler. She sleeps in my bed, at my invitation – naughty, I know, but hey, there are worse things!

Medicinal cannabis is now being prescribed in the UK, on special licence, to children suffering from epilepsy. It is expected the reforms will be through government by late autumn. How different things could have been for us if this had been the case five years ago. This has been a personal battle for me, with many letters written to MPs and pressure groups. I am so glad-hearted for all those who will benefit, and I eagerly await its use for MS, Parkinson's and cancer, amongst many other diseases and conditions.

I am 'healthy'; my cancer has not returned, despite my best efforts with alcohol and cigarettes. My womb biopsies were clear. However, my self-medication with these substances continues. Time will tell, and I swing between caring a lot and trying to be 'good', and depression and anxiety states where I just don't care enough.

I sent the majority of the oil Jasper and I made out into the world, to those who had pressing need for it.

Diary, 1st August 2018

I approach my fifty-second birthday, and I am fearful –
only eight years until I am sixty! Will I make it, and if so,
what will life be like? I still think of death every day, either

by cancer or my own hand; maybe, though, that is exactly the same. It's inevitable, death, the only thing we can all be sure of. But it looms large and I know if I continue to dwell on it, it will come sooner than is maybe necessary.

I await the return of hope, as I await the dying. Hope is key; without it we are lost. I am lost.

I hope for enduring friendships that don't need conditions. I hope for someone to physically love me, tenderly and with care, and to be a companion to my strange self; maybe not every day, maybe not in my home, maybe just a steady partner to share the ups and downs of this life.

I hope to find my muse again, to write and sing and play in the sun. I hope to keep hoping.

Onward ho.

I seem to have accepted my widowhood and my sadness.

I have learnt there is no getting through or past or over the loss of someone it's inconceivable to live without. There is only an acceptance to live alongside it, to create spaces for it to be a sacred and precious thing to hold near.

March 2019, Peebles

I have struggled to really complete this memoir, to lay it to bed; to be finished with delving into memory and diaries and trying to find answers to unsolvable questions. Should I send it away to a publisher? I was truly stuck and couldn't figure what was going on, why wasn't it done? Would it never be done? It wasn't as if I was working on it. It just sat there; a big, dark lump of unfinishedness. A reflection of my apathy. I had no inspiration in any direction. I gave up. I had lost the trust in intuitive creativeness which understands when it's not complete. It turns out there was more, and I deeply needed to end it with an optimism that was heartfelt and true; not a hopeful optimism that just wings it with fingers crossed, but a new truth for me.

Twenty eighteen turned out to be the year of nothing. However, it was a busy year in terms of the Jasper King Trust charity fundraising and good work achieved for families in need of respite; we sent four families to Harvest Moon in East Lothian, and made a difference to them in their coping. Our fundraising efforts were mighty and included Jaspers best friend Dave completing a journey from Lands End to John O Groats by bicycle; a huge achievement.

Lucy and Mick gave their time and skills to a project building a kitchen room on the side of the caravan on Eigg. They completed it in five days. In fifty hours, without plans, they broke ground, problem solved, worked with humour and diligence, and created a beautiful wooden Sharashack for me to cook, live, and entertain in. The six-by-eight-foot caravan became my cosy bedroom. It was a long hoped for dream and it was hugely aided by Damian, who ordered and stored the build materials for us.

Twenty Eighteen was busy in terms of me having an elderly stalker who helped wreck my head and depleted my confidence and energy further. A kindness from me was taken, twisted and abused, and this left me shaken and scared and highlighted just how isolated I felt. He emailed me repeatedly; sometimes several times a day, becoming increasingly odd and emotionally demanding. This came to a head early in May, as my dear old Grandma Anne passed away, at the grand old age of one hundred and five. She and I were very close and visiting her was very much part of my weekly routine. Jasper and she had always laughed together and he had a cheeky way with her that she loved; she would twinkle her green eyes at him and say; "Put your arm around me Jasper". Grandmas passing was another broken connection, another big shift. I was having major panic attacks again, I stopped going into college, where I was sitting end of course exams, because the attacks were happening there too. I felt horribly out of control and vulnerable. The stalker was dealt with eventually by the JKT board members who formed a protective virtual wall around me, so he could no longer contact me and feed off my uncertainty and fear. All his emails went directly to Sue and she contacted me if she thought I needed to be aware or concerned. I couldn't face reporting him to the police; by this time I was pretty much housebound with depression.

I hit rock bottom in late August 2018, while on Eigg, and realised I needed help, urgently. I rang my GP and headed back to Edinburgh to finally stand and face myself.

It was a busy year for moving again; having sunk so far into depression I had no choice but to return and live with my parents. I had lost any care for myself, only the dog kept me moving enough to stay in the world, and I was terrified of being alone and what I may do to myself. It had been thirty years since our family had shared a home and was a huge challenge for us all. There was a nightmare eight weeks of frantically giving away my possessions, living at my parents', and travelling into Edinburgh to try and empty the flat before my lease ran out. I would arrive full of good intentions, walk in, and become pretty much immediately overwhelmed, move a couple of things to the car and leave again. It was utterly exhausting. Bless Ali, my lovely pal, for all his trooping up and down the three flights of stairs for me, loading my car. I spent weeks sadly trying to rehome precious furniture. It couldn't go back to the parents' garage! It was a busy year for a brand-new life, setting up in a rented, sunny, ground-floor flat in Peebles, with a wee front garden. A hard move with no help with decorating or shifting the boxes out of the garage. I felt I had used up all my goodwill with friends; I was still deeply isolated by depression. I paid some fellows to move the big stuff; I somehow did the rest.

It was an especially busy year with my new companion, my love, my best friend: my own little long-short dog, Frida Kahlo; Jack Russell x Collie x Whippet?

However, at a deep level I felt nothing at best throughout this year; at worst it was a dark year of sluggish brain, panic attacks, constant anxiety, never having enough money. I was too unwell physically to manage the three flights of stairs up to the flat. I was worrying about the future and ruminating on the past. I had poor eating habits, was drinking heavily and smoking alongside my self-made social isolation, and at all times I was accompanied by the darkest thoughts, each running incessantly to the seemingly natural conclusion of suicide or how to bring about my accidental death.

Apparently, it is still called a nervous breakdown. I named it, in disbelieving whispers to myself. The GP diagnosed it. At least I had a name for it. I said to people, "I have had a nervous breakdown. I am very unwell." It was like speaking through a fog. I could hear myself, but I wasn't present. Still, it's like severe depression; if you've not been there, how can you know what it is like? It wasn't like a breaking down, though; that implies something suddenly stopping, and this was so slow it was imperceptible. I didn't even know I had been falling into it for many months, years, until I was suddenly already there, in the night, on Eigg, in the water, in the wave, so cold, and I am falling.

The GP was great. My folks were great. My daughter was great. Pals were great. The dog was great. Everyone was great, and everything was flawed by the constant thoughts of an ending to life, and the urgent need to leave Edinburgh, and all it had come to represent to me.

Frida and I settled as well as we could at my folks' in Peebles; we made our room into a nest and let them take care of us for a while – love, company and food provided. I slept a lot and I also drifted round the house, hollow-eyed, hoping to find the missing parts of myself.

I immediately began walking the dog around the paths of my younger self, my teenage years, my school years, my childhood, along the mighty River Tweed and up around the hills and woods. Over the next few months I found comfort in the sublime that I desperately needed. Initially the river walks would be filled with thoughts of jumping in the water, daydreams of how and where would be best to float away. I'd have to take the dog with me, somehow make it look as though she had gone in and I'd gone in after her; it would have to look like an accident. I would walk the woods imagining myself swinging from the rope swings. Imagining the horror of the person who found me.

I had gone back to the start, somewhere I never thought I could live again, in the hope of a new beginning. The dog kept me moving and looking outward, and her antics began to cut through the mist. The new pill dosage (forty milligrams) started to work and the fog began to clear. My energy came back, and the dark thoughts, the ones that were ever present and ever dangerous, receded. It was a relief to slowly feel some clarity return and, importantly, to be able to look ahead and make plans so that life resumed in some way. To be able to look back and see how close to the void I had been for a long time. So many lessons learned. I quit smoking again; maybe smoking was a way of punishing myself for all the things I felt I had done wrong while Jasper was sick. These thoughts require deeper introspection, when I finally get my referral through from the psychiatrist I have seen at the GP's request. I am awaiting a programme of psychodynamic therapy, a year or more of talking sessions aimed at finding out why I react to depression the way I do, to look at my earlier life and see where these coping mechanisms began.

Unfortunately, it seems that antidepressants work for a while, but after a month or so of feeling better, the up affects wear off and I am back to depression and numbness. This frightens me as I don't know how I will ever come off them. The withdrawal when I miss a dose is profound; cramps in my legs and arms, a feeling of a vice around my temples, jaws and neck, and loud cracks and pops in my ears. I think I am crazy; however, BBC Radio 4 have been running an excellent programme about long term use of antidepressants and the effects I am experiencing are widely reported by users. Feedback from patients on long term use, is only just beginning to be acknowledged, collated and reported on. Frida is my constant companion and I can attribute her companionship, love and loyalty to a large part of my recovery. She has assuaged the dreadful loneliness; she is someone to pour love onto and to set routines by. She makes me laugh and she keeps me warm at night; my sleepwalking and night terrors have abated. Instead of being afraid to go to bed, because it's empty and cold, and some night staying on the couch till 4am, or even just sleeping there, I am glad to go to bed early and cuddle her. I love her deeply and am grateful every day to have her with me.

Oranges and snow

In February 2019, I was recovering from yet another spontaneous broken rib. I had been diagnosed with osteoporosis in 2017 after ten broken ribs and a broken wrist, all in under five years, and my irradiated chest wall was a constant source of pain and new rib fractures. I desperately needed some sunshine and vitamin D. I took a flight to Spain to go and stay with a friend whom I had met only briefly in Edinburgh, but with whom I shared many friends and a passion for politics. Brexit was now the absolute disaster we had all feared it would be. We stood on the brink of being disconnected, cut off from our European friends, and our freedom to roam and work in the EU was about to be curtailed. I wanted to go before I couldn't, so I booked a cheap flight, left the dog with my parents and set off for ten days in the Andalusian sunshine.

What a tonic; the sun, the clean air, the different way of life. People to laugh with. I realised how deep my depression still was. Amanda and I got on very well indeed, both enjoying big chats and *vino tinto*. She and her husband had only been there six months and were busy renovating a *finca* with a swimming pool to let out to tourists.

I was charmed by the *fincas'* that filled the hillsides of the *campo*; white houses with wide terraces, set on steep valleys filled with trees growing oranges, lemons, olives, almonds and avocados. So much lovely food, all growing right there on the doorstep, and way behind and up in the distance the white capped Sierras de Tejeda mountains; the highlands. Oranges and snow. The other views down the valleys led the eye to the glittering Mediterranean, and in the evenings, as dusk fell, Africa's shores would come hazily into view. It was magical.

I flippantly said to Amanda, "Where shall I put my yurt?"

She laughed and said, "Wherever you like, there's plenty room." This joke became a new reality over the time I was there.

I left feeling very happy; there is a new way. I will go back in January 2020, if I can get into the country. I have already rented the *finca* for a month. I will bring friends with me to clear the ground, lay decking; I will buy a yurt (expensive) and create a self-contained camping area with yurt, solar panels, kitchen and shower room, eco toilet and a terrace for dining, along with a wildlife garden. This will take a while to bring to fruition, but it holds one of the keys to my future. The yurt will earn money for both myself and Amanda during the summer months, and in the winter Frida and I can live there rent free. (If she can leave the UK – so many ifs...)

The beginning...

As I approach Jasper's fourth anniversary and seven years since this all began, I can finally look ahead, truly, and see a new life of possibilities. There is forward motion; after four years of wondering how to approach the horror that Jaspers ashes have represented to me, he is now resting in a beautiful ceramic urn, made by our friend Miche, and it is shaped exactly like his juggling club, which I took to her workshop back in 2016.

Sue, Dave, Marion and I will return to Eigg at mid-summer and we will bury him, next to the caravan, under an apple tree gifted by Sarah and Ian. Jasper will also be with us on Laig Bay over the longest day, as the tide comes in, and his ashes will be taken by the waves to far flung places. I feel at peace making this decision; he will always be at the caravan, on Laig Bay and in our oceans.

Cannabis oil played a huge part in our travels with cancer; I do not regret any of the decisions we made regarding its use, growing our own supply and making our oil. In 2019, I can now buy CBD oil at my local chemist or go to a specialist shop, where I can purchase a wide range of oils and take advice on how they might aid my health. I have tried a few, but to be honest, I feel the zero content of THC has an impact on efficacy.

I have also tasted iso in some of shop bought oils and I wonder how the industry is regulated. I am frustrated at the legislation which criminalises cannabis users; I continue to campaign for a broader understanding of this natural plant and its many uses.

Medicinal cannabis prescriptions rely on a sympathetic GP, and a special license from the Home Office. There are still parents with epileptic children, fighting for its use to reduce the frequency of fits they have per day. Cancer, MS and Parkinson's sufferers are still awaiting life changing legislation; cannabis oil has been shown to ease symptoms in these and other diseases. In the meantime, the UK now exports and grows seventy percent of the world's medicinal cannabis. There is so much wrong with this dichotomy; UK illegality of use versus UK production for export, but that's another story.

I think depression will always play a part; it's always there, a background hum. There will be days of missing and longing, leaning into the hug that isn't there, and there will always be the need to say his name out loud. Time has healed some of the deep wounds; on my heart, soul and my psyche, and has also shifted perspectives. I have acceptance. I have learned to be without Jasper here in the physical world. I have found that solo living, while having it challenges, also suits me. Leaving Edinburgh has been such a positive move. I need green spaces and natures beauty and I can see the sunlight again; my dog, my kitchen, my garden, and the countryside, continue to soothe me. I am hopeful and much happier.

If I could send my younger self a letter, a 'map' of bereavement, I would say the following; let it take you when the waves hit. Lay down if you must. Hold on tight to the thoughts of better days to come. Let children and friends distract you. Plan for the big days – be busy if you can. Numbness is your way of coping; particularly when you're not coping. There is no wrong way to feel. Honour the dead and know they are with us every day, some days much more than others. I believe they are now energy and can be found anywhere there is life, anywhere you need to look. Take time to be by yourself, learn to live quietly and try to find a peace within you. Take the pills if they are needed but be wise to their payload. Grief has an ebb and flow, it changes over time, but it will always be part of our journey, each one a different path, but all sharing many commonalities of love, isolation, fear, panic, unbearable grief, physical pain, PTSD, depression, insomnia, hopelessness, and moments of utter clarity and madness.

Time goes by; it's relentless, and the moments of being OK get longer and the moments of not being OK get less sharp; but there are no straight lines, no fast forward, and there is no map.

And in time, there will be a return of light and joy.

I think Jasper would very much approve of my decision to leave the UK, at least over winter, just as we had planned to do way back when, with our Australian visas. He would encourage me to keep moving, to look after my bones, to feed my nomadic soul, and to live in a place where the sun shines.

He asked me, not long before he died, to keep my heart open and to carry on hoping; he understood living without hope is impossible, and that somewhere in the future, the sun will shine through.

Good luck, fellow travellers.

The Infinite Shades of Missing

Here inside these nuances of missing,
Which are infinite in their shades;
In troughs and swells and sideswipes
And sometimes just clean greys.

Heart-held precious moments,
Disconnected in our times,
I'm in the Birnam ballroom,
Your hands, your heart, your eyes in mine.

In bursts of sun-filled certainty,
Dragonflies and cow parsley.
Your head thrown back in laughter
And your many shades of red.

The missing never seems to sleep,
It's in all the endless places.
Sometimes clear, pure despair,
And I feel you in intangible embraces.

Yesterday, today, tomorrow;
Thereafter, hereafter – ever after.
A part of me has gone on with you,
And part of you remains with me. Please stay.

In madness and in learning,
In the loneliness of alone,
In blue coats and Roman noses,
In stoical living and in cooking for one.

In drinking in the afternoon and smoking dreadful fags;
In a quiet, slow suicide.
In finding strength where there is fear.
And in living in the moment, for a moment.

In twisted dreams and night terrors,
And futile rumination.
In seeing the leaving hours on constant replay;
A background buzz, a daily station.

In watching seasons pass,
Spring to spring – a year!
I feel the tribe soothing at my back,
Your name, your name, but you're not here. Stay.

In the pencil that you sharpened,
And your clothes and shoes I cannot give away.
In your old, broken, not-much-used tools and golfing tees.
There are parts of you that stay.

I inhabit the whole of our bed,
But in the night awake to find myself
Curled around the shape of you.

I make a mess in our car,
And smile at how you would approve.

In aimless walking and aimless longing,
And in all the spaces in between.
How come, if you are in everything,
You are not here? Stay.

In the 'I am a cuckoo' calls and the white magnolia flower.
In the forget-me-nots and the roses,
And the vastness of the endless hours.
Stay.

In Hale-Bopp's blazing trail,
And the soaring of the hawk.
And the beach walks and the two steps.
And the endless talk, talk, talk,
Of recovery.

In the zephyrs and the floating winds,
And the just being sat sitted.
And the holding hands and holding toes,
And the myriad things we never admitted.

In your triangle and your cowbell,
Your clogs, clubs and fire torches.
In your beautiful tenor uke,
And all the Chipolata costumes.

In the FHB and WTF and LOFL.
The turns of your wrists and your crooked smile.
And the missing, the missed, the mist.
Stay.

In the late-night curries
And "Don't cook the spoon."
And "I love you anyways."
All the "bits and stuffs and pieces".
And... the TV sport on Sunday's.

Stay.